Swara Yoga

The Indian Science of Right Timing

TOMER WEISS

SWARA YOGA: The Indian Science of Right Timing

First Edition: 2026

Editor: Traci Rose Rider
Cover and Interior Design: Tomer Weiss
ISBN: 978-965-93344-0-7

Practice Disclaimer: The information in this book is for educational and informational purposes only. Swara Yoga and somatic practices involve rhythmic breathing and physical awareness. Please consult with a healthcare professional before beginning any new respiratory or physical program. The author and publisher disclaim any liability for injuries or loss in connection with the practices and advice contained in this book.

Published by: Shivoham Press
[www.integraldepth.com/books]

For my friends:

Ron, who has been my Vajra support along the way;
Yoav, who first sparked my interest in Svara;
Itay and Itay, who introduced me to the world of yoga
more than twenty-five years ago and have walked
this path alongside me since;
Boaz, who remains close even when continents away;
Fraser, who agreed to take some of the photos;
and last but not least-
Daniel, who bought me my first yoga books
and opened the door for me to deepen my studies.

May this book find you
at the right time.

Table of Contents

Introduction
Listening to the Breath of Time

Breath meditation is perhaps the most widely practiced form of meditation on the planet. We follow the breath as it moves in and out of the body. Yet within this familiar practice, the breath hides a quiet rhythm we rarely notice, a rhythm that profoundly shapes our lives. At times the breath flows more freely through the right nostril, at other times through the left. It subtly alternates in cycles throughout the day and night, and influences mood, focus, brain function, and the way we act in the world.

Long before modern physiology described this pattern, Indian yogis understood it well. They called it *svara* — the "sound" or "flow" of the breath — and saw in it the same forces that move the sun and the moon, stir the tides, and guide the seasons.

To these yogis, breath was not just a bodily process but a mirror of the cosmic order, a living bridge between inner and outer nature. They chose to live in alignment with this rhythm, carefully timing their actions with the right flow, and discovering a way of life with less friction and more easeful flow.

A Life Out of Rhythm

Today, most of us live out of tune with this rhythm. We wake to an alarm, eat by the clock, and sleep only when the screen goes dark. on some level, you probably already sense this and recognize the strain that arises from overriding your natural biological clock.

Modern life is plagued by sleep disturbances, hormonal imbalances, nervous tension, and chronic fatigue — conditions that often begin to improve when we realign with the natural cycles of day and night. Yet Svara Yoga suggests that this circadian rhythm is just one layer. It points to a more intricate inner clock, one that influences not only how we rest but also how each and every action unfolds.

If your life feels like an ongoing struggle — as if your engine is running at full throttle yet you're not truly moving forward — chances are you're living out of step with your inner rhythm. When efforts that should have worked" falter for no obvious reason, it may simply be a matter of timing: your actions weren't in harmony with the cycles of time.

This book is an invitation to return to that rhythm. By learning to listen and to align with the cycles of your own breath, you will explore how to time your actions so they are supported rather than obstructed, and how to move toward the results you truly want with greater clarity, ease, and flow.

The Promise of Svara Yoga

Svara Yoga is the science of living in rhythm. It teaches us to read the language of the breath and to act in harmony with its cycles: when to move outward and when to turn inward, when to speak and when to remain silent, when to initiate and when to rest.

Imagine applying for a job when the company isn't hiring — your application sinks to the bottom of the pile. Or asking someone on a date just after they've started a new relationship. In the same way, planting seeds in the peak of summer, months before the rains arrive, ignores the simple truth that timing shapes outcomes.

Every action has a moment that amplifies its potential. With the wisdom of Svara yoga, our breath becomes a kind of inner compass, orienting us with the natural cycles of day and night, the elements, the seasons, and the subtle shifts in the energies of consciousness itself. It teaches us how to recognize the right time for each action so that what we do is supported, rather than opposed, by the larger rhythm of life.

My Experiences with the Svara

I first encountered Svara Yoga in 2005, when I read Swami Sivananda's book on the subject. At the time it felt esoteric, abstract, and somewhat disconnected from my everyday life. I doubted its scientific validity and didn't pursue it.

Years later, during a period of significant life challenges, I began to notice a striking difference between my experience and the experiences of some people around me. Life seemed to unfold with more ease. Things would "fall into place" with relatively little effort, while I often felt I had to struggle — often failing despite my best efforts.

In 2019, everything shifted. While developing a treatment modality for migraine headaches, which included a technique of directing the breath through the left nostril at first signs of an attack, I came across the work of David Shannahoff-Khalsa. His research showed that manipulating the nostril flow could profoundly influence physiology, cognition, and psychology, offering solid medical confirmation that the Svara can shape both mental and physical states.

This was the first solid medical confirmation that the Svara could impact mental and physical states which opened for me the door for deeper exploration.

I began not only to align my life with these teachings — but also to research them intensively. I sought out ancient texts, clinical reports, and spiritual insights. In doing so, I not only deepened my understanding, but uncovered source material never before brought forth in this way.

In this book, I've tried to preserve the depth and nuance of the traditional teachings while translating them into a language modern readers can grasp. My aim is to keep the integrity of the tradition intact while showing that this isn't just an Indian concept — it's a universal human truth.

What You Will Discover

In these pages, you will:

- Learn how the alternating breath relates to the brain hemispheres, the autonomic nervous system, and the dual currents of prāṇa known as *Iḍā* and *Piṅgalā.*
- Explore how the five elements (*tattvas*) and the planetary hours influence your energy and perception throughout the day.
- Study the ancient techniques of *trāṭaka*, *mudrā*, and breath observation to recognize which *svara* is active at any given moment.
- Understand how to align your daily actions — from decision-making to creative work — with the flow of breath and time.
- See how these teachings correspond with findings in modern science, psychology, and chronobiology.
- Learn how to apply this knowledge to support your own spiritual evolution.

This is not a theoretical study but a lived, practical system for experiencing life as a rhythmic field of intelligence — where breath, mind, and cosmos move as one.

How to Read This Book

This book is not meant to be rushed or understood only with the intellect. It is meant to be breathed.

I have tried to keep the content as accessible as possible while honoring both the science and the tradition. You'll find simple explanations alongside deeper explorations of philosophy and research, and if a section ever feels too dense, you can skip it and still stay connected to the heart of the work.

When I teach, I try to offer students a direct experience *before* anything is explained. This way, the insight emerges from their own perception, rather from borrowed concepts. The chapters in this book are structured in the same way, with exercises and meditations to support that process and help you do the same.

Treat each chapter as an experiment. As you read, let the pages become instructions that you carry into your body: try the meditations, feel what I describe, and only then return to the philosophical explanations to refine and deepen your understanding.

I invite you to study this book slowly. The capacity to perceive the svara, in all its subtlety, develops with practice. What may feel like imagination at first will, with time, becomes clear, grounded, and unmistakably real.

This shift is born of a deep realignment that cannot be rushed, so let the teachings reshape you at their own pace. Let time breathe with you.

As you move through the chapters, pause now and then. Feel the air move through your nostrils, notice which side flows more freely, and let this simple awareness accompany you as a quiet thread through your reading.

Because *Svara Yoga* is not only something you learn, it's something you begin to *live*. And when you do, time itself begins to breathe with you.

PART I: UNDERSTANDING SVARA YOGA

Chapter 1
The Cycles Of Nature

Nature's Cycles and the Myths That Explained Them

Since time immemorial, mankind has been captivated by the cyclical patterns of nature. People noticed the shifting of the seasons and how this affected the plants and animals around them. The sun's daily arc across the sky and how this daily journey shifted throughout the year. The moon's waxing and waning, the ebb and fall of the tides and the celestial dance of the planets. All these have steered our curiosity. These phenomena have been immortalized in our collective memory through myths and stories, serving as a testament to our enduring fascination with them.

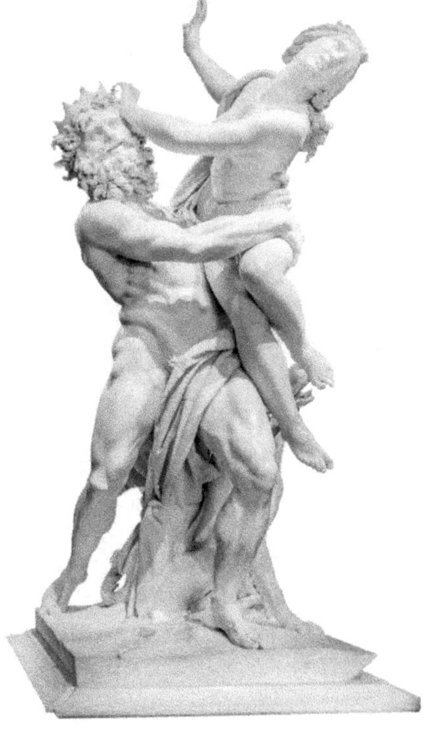

Consider the Greek myth of Persephone and Hades. Persephone, daughter of Demeter, goddess of harvest, represents vegetation and the flourishing of life, while Hades, god of the underworld, embodies death and the hidden, mysterious aspects of existence. One day, while gathering flowers in a meadow, Persephone is abducted by Hades, and, with Zeus' consent, taken to the underworld as his queen. Demeter's grief over her lost daughter leads her to withdraw from her duties as the guardian of agriculture, leading to famine on Earth. Zeus eventually intervenes, negotiating Persephone's return to the surface. However, because Persephone has eaten a pomegranate seed in the underworld, she must spend a part of each year below and part above. Persephone's journey symbolizes and explains the changes our world goes through in the seasons. Her descent corresponds to winter, when life retreats and the land appears barren, and her return to the surface heralds spring, renewal, and the reawakening of life and vegetation.

Long before humanity developed modern science, such myths and spiritual philosophies served as living models of reality. By recognizing which stories were central to a culture, we can sense what that culture was trying to understand, because people tell stories about the things that matter to them. These stories reflect our primal need: to explain and predict the world around us so that it feels less threatening and unknown. An unpredictable world is a frightening and dangerous world; but through explaining it and understanding how it operates, some of this fear is alleviated. And so humanity has always tried to explain and understand what causes events to unfold in the world around us.

Imagine the fear people must have felt when facing the disappearance of the sun in a solar eclipse. Next to the unknown, the dark was the scariest thing for ancient humanity. The dark meant death. Upon seeing a solar eclipse, people believed the world might end or that some great malevolent force was descending upon them. Stories became a way to soften that terror. Explaining what was happening—and trusting that the process would be reversed—offered reassurance and even a sense that humans could participate in mending the situation. Different cultures responded in vivid, symbolic ways. In Colombia people shouted out to the heavens, promising to work harder and correct their actions, while among the Chipewa, fear drove warriors to shoot flaming arrows into the sky in a desperate bid to rekindle the sun. Meanwhile, in parts of Peru, tribes also sent fire into the sky, but with a different motive: they believed a beast was attacking the sun and hoped the flames would drive it away. Across traditions, the eclipse's eerie atmosphere stirred humanity into diverse rituals, prayers, and actions throughout history.

Having a story was far more comforting than having no explanation at all. Ancient humanity thus used myths to weave meaning around the cycles of nature so that people could feel a measure of predictability and control in an unpredictable world. The waxing and waning of the moon, for example, was attributed in the Hindu tradition to a curse placed on the moon god Chandra for his infatuation with the 27 celestial nymphs, while among the Navajo, the moon was seen as a warrior who gained strength as the moon waxed and weakened as it waned.

Over time, people noticed how these cycles affected their own lives directly. They watches animals hibernate, traced the migrations of various creatures they hunted, and noticed how trees lost their leaves in winter and bore fruits again in spring. Most of all, humanity noticed how these rhythms governed the availability of food. Once people transitioned from the nomadic hunting and gathering to agriculture, recognizing seasonal patterns became essential for survival. This shift called for an intimate understanding of when to plant, tend, and harvest, and from this need, an art of right timing emerged. By observing which stars rose with the sun, people could tell which season was beginning and choose the right course of action for the months ahead.

From Sky to Self: Cycles in the Body

In time, attention turned from the sky to the body, and people began to notice inner cycles as clearly as outer ones. The first to stand out was likely the menstrual cycle, which closely mirrors the cycle of the moon, both being around 28-29 days. Archaeologists have found a 22,000-year-old bone known as the Ishango bone in the present-day Democratic

Republic of Congo, marked with tally lines that follow a 28-day pattern, suggesting it was an early menstrual tracker. Humanity also recognized the link between the menstrual cycle and the birth of children, and many ancient cultures believed that uterine blood somehow congealed and transformed into the fetus and, eventually, the child. From this, humanity understood that in the same way that there is a right time for planting seed in the Earth, there was a right time for the human seed to take root in the womb. The rhythms of fertility became another expression of the same wisdom of timing that governed agriculture and the seasons.

Besides menstruation and the great arc of life from birth to death, other cycles revealed themselves. The cycle of sleep that draws us to rest in the evening and back to wakefulness in the morning, and the cycle of breath, continually entering and leaving the body, changing in quality and depth throughout the day. Many additional biological cycles were noticed as well: the body becoming warmer or cooler, more stiff or more flexible, hungry and then satiated, growing tall and gradually shrinking with age, and many more. All of these patterns hinted that the same cyclical intelligence shaping the heavens is also at work within the human body.

The Art of Right Timing

Drawing from their experience with agriculture, ancient people came to a simple yet powerful understanding: human activities flourish when they are aligned with both the outer cycles of nature and the inner cycles of the body. Synchronizing with these rhythms was seen as a way to find the path of least resistance, like catching the wind in a sail at just the right moment, or letting a boat move with the flow of the river rather than against it.

Over time, this insight evolved into guidelines for living. These were not only about when to plant and when to harvest, but also when to marry, when to embark on journeys, and when to begin constructing a new home. These were all rooted in the belief that acting at the right time invites favorable results, while acting out of sync with these rhythms can hinder fruition. Thus, in search of ways to control their destiny, cultures looked for the best time to take an action.

When there were few other means of influencing destiny, choosing the most auspicious moment became its own art. I'm sure that you probably recognize this in your daily life: approaching someone at the right moment can open doors, while approaching the same person with the same request but in an importune moment might not get you what you want.

The art of right timing applies as much to human relationships as it does the cycles of nature. It helps to clarify not only when to take actions and when to pause, but also which moments naturally support what actions.

Moreover, for many cultures, this approach was not just about practical wisdom. It expressed a profound recognition of the interconnectedness between humans and their environment. To move in harmony with the cycles of the cosmos was to enter a spiritual current of energy, a flow that linked human life to the divine.

By honoring these cycles, people sought both physical well-being and spiritual harmony. Timing became the key to fruition, pointing to a profound connection between human existence and the broader cycles of nature.

In this book, we are going to study about the various cycles of ancient nature, mainly through the lens of the Indian tradition, especially those related to Svara. Svara means "breath": the breath of nature and its cycles, and the breath that moves in and out of our nostrils. We will explore the Svara of the elements and how they ebb and flow, the rhythms of qi in Chinese medicine, and of *prāṇa* in Ayurveda. And we will learn how these patterns relate to astrology, planetary hours, and the magical hours of the Western esoteric tradition. A central question throughout will be which actions are best supported by which Svara and timeframe. In other words, how to recognize, in practice, the right time for each kind of movement.

This teaching is based on traditional sources, presenting the spiritual theory behind this science while also relating it to modern scientific research and understanding. We'll explore the ancient wisdom and the scientific basis underlying these discoveries. Through understanding all this, you will be able to know when to take what action to make the most of your life. But before we can work with these cycles, we need to understand what Svara Yoga actually is. So let's strip away the complexity and get to the essence—in the next chapter, a ten-minute read, you'll understand the core principles that took ancient yogis' lifetimes to master.

Chapter 2
Svara Yoga Explained in 10 Minutes

So what exactly is Svara Yoga? Svara Yoga is the Indian science of right timing: aligning one's actions with the flow of energies in the body and in the universe to move with the flow of life, meet less resistance, and receive maximum return on our efforts. In Sanskrit, *svara* means the sound or flow of one's own breath, and *yoga* means union, so *Svara Yoga* is the path of union through one's own breath—through listening to, and observing, our breath. It invites us either to adjust our actions based on our breath, or to adjust the breath according to the actions or outcomes we want to achieve.

Here, *svara* is the flow, the rhythm—not only of our physical breath, but also of our subtle energetic breath and the breath-like cycles of nature. The central idea is that nature undergoes certain cycles and that our human body undergoes cycles that correspond to these. When the inner and outer rhythms are aligned, actions tend to succeed more easily. When the two cycles are misaligned, our actions are not as effective. So in the overarching scheme, Svara Yoga teaches us about these cycles of nature and how to live in harmony with them. It shows how to recognize which cycle of nature is currently active, which phase in that cycle best supports a given action, and which phase of our internal cycle is best suited to that action. From there, practice becomes an art of alignment: bringing together the natural cycle, the internal cycle, and our chosen action. When we align all three, the likelihood of achieving what we intend increases greatly, even exponentially.

Now, the cycles of nature cannot be changed; they can only be observed and met. Quite a few of the body's cycles also run automatically and cannot easily be shifted. But there is one rhythm we influence directly and skillfully: the pattern of our breathing. This is why a lot of the knowledge given in Svara Yoga teaches us how to modify this cycle to bring us success.

But although a significant portion of Svara Yoga focuses on how to work with this modifiable cycle of the breath, it should not be confused with *Pranayama*, the Indian practice of controlling the breath, or with such breath-awareness practices such as the Buddhist meditation of *Anapanasati*. While Pranayama works to control or redirect *prāṇa*, and while Anapanasati emphasizes the uninterrupted and non-analytical observation of the breath. Svara Yoga, by contrast, centers on the *analysis* of the breath and using the knowledge gained by this analysis to decode the inner rhythms operating in the body in order to achieve specific, desired effects.

Exercise 1: Experience the Svara

Sit in a comfortable position and notice your breath as it moves in and out through your nostrils. Don't try to change the flow of the air—simply notice how the breath comes in and out of the nostrils. Notice whether the airflow feels equal in both nostrils, or if one nostril seems a little clearer while the other feels slightly more blocked.

If you're not sure, gently close one of your nostrils—left or right—and breathe only through the unblocked nostril for a few moments, sensing how easy or difficult the air moves there. Now switch sides, closing this nostril and breathing through the one that was previously blocked, and notice the difference in effort and sensation. The breath will most likely flow more strongly though one rather than the other.

Now release both nostrils and rest the back of your hand just beneath them. As you breathe in and out, feel where the air coming out of one nostril is stronger. The side where you sense more airflow is your predominant nostril in this moment. There's always one nostril that is a little more open, a little more free. If you check again in about 90 minutes, you will almost certainly find that the dominant side has switched. Curious, no?

There are several ways to explain why this happens. Modern medicine offers physiological reasons, and traditional Indian teachings describe it in terms of subtle energy, which we will explore in more depth. According to the science of Svara Yoga, when we are breathing mainly through one nostril, the life-force energy—termed *prāṇa*—is flowing in our being in a particular way, and when the dominant nostril changes, the flow and quality of that prāṇa energy shifts as well.

The Theory Behind Svara

According to Svara Yoga, there are three energy channels, or *nāḍīs*, through which this breath can flow. The *Iḍā nāḍī*, which is connected with the left nostril; the *Piṅgalā nāḍī*, connected to the right nostril; and the *Suṣumnā nāḍī*, in which the breath is experienced as neither predominantly left or right. Each pattern of flow has a distinct influence on physiology, how we feel, how we think, how we perceive the world, and how we act in it.

Now this is already quite intuitive on one level, but the Indian tradition goes a step further by suggesting that certain actions are more likely to succeed when performed under a specific flow—through one nostril rather than the other. In other words, the state of the breath is not only a reflection of inner conditions, but also a guide to the most supportive timing for what you choose to do.

So the science of Svara Yoga therefore maps which kinds of actions are best undertaken when we're breathing through the right or left nostril, and which actions we should avoid. The emphasis is on *naturally* breathing through your nostrils, not proactively closing one. In other words, Svara Yoga teaches that certain actions performed while the breath flows predominantly through the left nostril are easier to perform, more fruitful, and bring greater results—while other actions should be done when the breath naturally flows through the right nostril.

The core of the Svara Yoga practice is how to synchronize our actions with this ongoing cycle of prāṇic energies moving through the body, expressed as breath going in through one nostril or the other. We will explore the spiritual explanations behind why Svara Yoga says this, but this book will also explore how modern neurology and psychology provide a complementary scientific basis for these ancient observations.. While some of these age-old observations could be dismissed as mystical speculation at first glance, a closer look through contemporary science explains why these traditional recommendations stand on firm ground. This will be the main focus of Svara Yoga.

There are additional aspects of Svara Yoga related to divination, that is, understanding how to read these cycles in order to foretell the future. We will touch upon these more briefly, since they are harder to verify scientifically and less central to everyday practice. When it comes to understanding the cycles of life and the timing of action, however, we can definitely bridge traditional insight and modern research to appreciate how both point toward the same subtle intelligence moving through breath and time.

Chapter 3
The Literature of Svara Yoga

Now that you have a sense of what Svara Yoga is and what it offers, you might be wondering: where does this knowledge come from?

Although the technical science of Svara Yoga was systemized in the Tantric period, its philosophical roots are far more ancient. The tradition stands upon a four-tiered lineage of knowledge: the Vedic Foundation, the Upanishadic Framework, Astrological writings and the Tantric Application.

1. The Vedic Foundation (1900-1500 BCE): Here, the Prāna is revered as the supreme, all-encompassing cosmic force, as seen in hymns like the *Prāna Sūkta,* which praise Prāna as the power behind the sun, moon, seasons, and life itself. These verses declare that when the right season comes and Prāna "calls" to the plants, everything on Earth becomes joyful.

"Homage, O Prāna, unto thee what time thou sendest down thy rain! ... When the due season hath arrived and Prāna shouteth to herbs, Then all is joyful, yea, each thing upon the surface of the earth".

and

"He is the Sun, he is the Moon. Prāna is called Prajāpati. ... On Prāna, past and future, yea, on Prāna everything depends".

2. **The Upanishadic Framework:** The Upanishads (c. 800-500 BCE) is where this cosmic Prāna is traced and mapped to the inner landscape of the body through internal, physiological pathways. Here we find the first

teachings on the subtle body that Svara Yoga relies on, including references in the *Bṛhadāraṇyaka Upaniṣad* to 72,000 nāḍīs filling the body. The *Taittirīya Upaniṣad* detailing of the *Prāṇamaya Kośa*, or the "body made of breath", and texts such as the *Maitrī Upaniṣad* that explain how the flow of prāṇa through the central channel, *suṣumnā*, presenting this inner ascent as the path to liberation.

3. Astrological and divinatory writings - By the late Vedic period (c. 1000–500 BCE), Indian seers had already developed a sophisticated system of lunar and solar reckoning—the *nakṣatra* (lunar mansion) calendar—rooted in ritual and agricultural cycles. When Hellenistic astrology entered India around the 2nd century BCE, it brought the twelve-sign zodiac (*rāśi*), planetary aspects, and horoscopic techniques, which Indian scholars—such as those behind the *Yavanajātaka* ("Sayings of the Greeks") and *Bṛhat Samhitā*—wove together with their native Vedic vision of cosmic order (*ṛta*) and karma. These helped shape *Jyotiṣa śāstra*, a uniquely Indian "science of light" linking celestial movements with moral and spiritual causality.

The *Bṛhat Samhitā* also preserved intricate techniques of omen-reading, including interpretations based on observing various bodily conditions like pimples or on momentary and seemingly random events like accidental touches. or the direction of approach of a person From here it was a short distance to apply similar predictive emphasis on the breath, which we see especially in the *Svara Cintāmaṇi.*

4. The Tantric Application: From around the 6th century CE onward, the *Tantras* who inherited this fully formed Vedic, Upanishadic, and astrological framework began developing it into an applied, practical discipline. Under the titles of Svara Yoga and *Kalachakra*, they shaped these ideas into methods that could be directly applied in practice, uniting cosmic cycles, breath, and time into a lived spiritual science.

The Svarodaya Śāstra

When speaking of the Svara Yoga literature or the *Svarodaya Śāstra*, most modern teachers, starting with Swāmī Śivānanda with his 1954 publication on the subject, primarily refer to two texts: The first, the ***Śiva Svarodaya*** (शवि स्‌वरोदय), is considered to be the foundational text of Svara Yoga. Its name means "The Rising of the Breath of Śiva", and it's written as a dialogue between Lord Śiva and his consort Pārvatī, where Śiva reveals the secrets of the breath to her.

When we look closely at this text, we find that it is somewhat disorganized: information jumps around, techniques are scattered, and sometimes the same topic appears in multiple places with slightly different details. This kind of structure is usually a sign that a text is a compilation of older material, which would suggest that this is not actually the earliest Svara Yoga text, but rather a later creation drawing from older sources.

The second text is the ***Svara Cintāmaṇi*** (स्‌वर चनि्तामणि), which means "The Wish-Fulfilling Gem of the Breath". While the *Śiva Svarodaya* has a more spiritual and philosophical tone, the *Svara Cintāmaṇi* is predominantly practical, almost like a professional manual. It is organized into chapters, each dedicated to specific types of questions a divinator or astrologer might receive from clients, with detailed instructions on how to determine the answer.

Both the texts are difficult to date with precision, though the *Śiva Svarodaya* was most likely written sometime between the 12th and 15th centuries, and the Cintāmaṇi being composed somewhat later. When I began to research the subject of Svara Yoga, I did not know the true original sources of this teaching. It is easy to be misled by traditional claims that the Shiva Svarodaya dates from somewhere between the 5th century BCE and the 5th century CE. As my research deepened, I found that many of the techniques taught in the *Śiva Svarodaya* appear in more organized or elaborated forms in other texts, such as the *Bardo Thödol* (the Tibetan Book of the Dead, 14th century), the *Kālacakra Tantra* (an 11th century Buddhist Tantra), the 7th century *Svacchanda Tantra*, and the *Kalottara Tantra*, possibly dating to the 6th century.

When trying to determine which text is original and which it the borrowing, one useful tool is to compare the richness and complexity of the information and teachings. For example, when comparing the *Śiva Svarodaya* with the *Bardo Thödol*, we see that certain techniques that receive only a single example in the *Śiva Svarodaya* are presented with five or ten variations in the Tibetan Book of the Dead. This could mean either that the shorter text is the earlier one, later elaborated into the richer teachings, or that it represents a fragment or compilation distilled from older, more extensive sources.

When we consider the brevity of the text and the fragmented way in which its teachings are presented, I have come to the conclusion that rather than being an original text, it appears more likely that this work is a later compilation that has, at times, lost parts of the earlier material on which it was based.

If the *Śiva Svarodaya* and the *Svara Cintāmaṇi* are therefore not the true origin of this teaching, the natural question arises: what is?

Indian Astrological Writings

The earliest origins of astrology trace back to ancient Mesopotamia, as early as 1900 BCE, where it focused mainly on interpreting celestial omens to predict events concerning the state and royalty (mundane astrology). In the Indian tradition, the first major astronomical text is the Vedanga Jyotisha, which centers on astronomical calculations and timekeeping used to determine the correct and auspicious moments for performing Vedic rituals and sacrifices.

Predictive astrology in India developed later, with the transmission of Hellenistic (Greek) astrological concepts. The first significant evidence of this exchange is the *Yavanajātaka* ("Sayings of the Greeks"), a translation of a Greek text into Sanskrit around the 2nd century CE, which introduced core elements of horoscopic astrology, including the 12 zodiac signs and the 12 astrological houses, that became the foundation of later Indian systems. Over time, these technical astrological teachings were woven together with existing philosophical and physiological ideas, especially the concept of prāṇa (breath or life force) described extensively in the Upanishads.

The Upanishads

Texts like the *Prashna Upanishad* describe how prāṇa arises from the Atman and divides into five forms to sustain all bodily functions, it also establishes that the individual breath acts as the living bridge between the individual body (*piṇḍa*) and the cosmic body (*brahmāṇḍa*), and describes the subtle cycle of the breath that underlies this relationship.

The Kalottara Tantra

The *Kālottara Tantra* ("Tantra of the Supreme Time"), probably from around the 7th century CE, is perhaps the first scripture to explicitly unite time (*kāla*), breath, and consciousness into a single principle. It teaches that each inhalation and exhalation echoes the waxing and waning of cosmic time, so that to observe one's breath is to watch the universe breathe, and that by aligning awareness with this inner rhythm, the yogin moves beyond the bondage of time itself and attains liberation. In this way, the *Kālottara* becomes one of the earliest sources to advocate observing the inner cycles of time present in the breath and to identify auspicious moments based on that observation, as well as the first to teach how through meditation one can modify the flow of time for oneself.

The *Svāccanda Tantra*

The *Svāccanda Tantra* ("Tantra of the Free One"), a Śaiva text from about the 7th century CE, offers another detailed teachings on using the breath as a means to liberation and on how cosmic cycles map to the breath. It dedicates its entire seventh chapter to teaching how the alternation of the breath between the nostrils corresponds to shifting mental and cosmic energies. From this, the core insight of Svara Yoga emerges clearly: by observing which nostril is dominant and how the flow changes, one can act in harmony with the larger natural forces.

The Tantrāloka

The *Tantrāloka* ("Light of the Tantras") by Abhinavagupta, written around the 10th–11th century, is one of the great syntheses of non-dual Śaiva philosophy and practice. Across its 37 chapters, it weaves ritual, yoga, and metaphysics into a single integrated vision of liberation. Although it never uses the term *Svara Yoga*, in chapter 6 Abhinavagupta comments on the *Svāccanda Tantra*, elaborating and refining its teachings.

The *Kālacakra Tantra*

The *Kālacakra Tantra*, or "Tantra of the Wheel of Time", an 11th-century Buddhist scripture, contains extensive teachings on time cycles, breath, and the movement of prāṇa through the body. Many of the techniques that appear briefly in the *Śiva Svarodaya* appear in more elaborate form in the *Kālacakra Tantra*, suggesting that Kālacakra may be the older, more developed text of these teachings. In this book, I will include information from the *Kālacakra Tantra* here and there, where it clarifies or deepens key points, and a dedicated chapter towards the end of the book will explore its vision of time and practice that go beyond the teachings of classical Svara Yoga.

The *Bardo Thödol* (Tibetan Book of the Dead)

The *Bardo Thödol*, more commonly known in English as the Tibetan Book of the Dead, contains remarkably similar teachings on predicting death through observing breath. Practices such as pressing on the eyes to perceive circles of light, and the shadow-gazing practice known as *Chāyopāsana*, appear there in much more detailed and elaborate forms than in the *Śiva Svarodaya*. This suggests a shared or intertwined stream of visionary and divinatory breath practices across Indian and Tibetan traditions.

The "renovation" of the *Śiva Svarodaya*

The *Śiva Svarodaya*, though not likely an entirely original text, does appear to be a kind of renovation or reworking of earlier teachings. It brings together the yogic teachings of the three nāḍīs, the three svaras (breath flow), and the cyclical alternation between the nostrils, and then applies this knowledge not primarily to liberation but to practical, worldly concerns. It focuses on mundane applications—globally inspired from the methods of astrologers and diviners—offering guidance for daily decisions, health, relationships, and success, all grounded in yogic science. In this way, the *Śiva Svarodaya* is both unique and genuinely innovative, translating subtle yogic insights into concrete advice for living well.

How This Book Uses the Source Texts

Throughout this book, I draw primarily from the ***Śiva Svarodaya*** for the core teachings of Svara Yoga, but I supplement this with the ***Svara Cintāmaṇi*** for additional prognostic techniques and specific applications. The ***Kālacakra Tantra*** provides a deeper context for understanding time cycles and elemental flows, while the ***Bardo Thödol*** offers more complete versions of certain visionary and death-related practices, particularly in the chapter on death signs. Where they genuinely expand or clarify the material, previously unpublished instructions from the ***Svaccanda*** and

***Kālottara Tantra*s** are also included, bringing to light dimensions of Svara Yoga that have rarely been accessible to modern practitioners.

When I reference these source texts in the chapters ahead, I'll name them explicitly so that you always know which tradition I'm drawing from. Sometimes I'll present the teachings exactly "as the text says", even when they do not fully align with modern understanding, because it is important to see what the tradition itself actually taught. After that, I will offer my own or a scientific interpretation, so you can better explore how these ancient insights might be understood and applied today.

Most modern books on Svara Yoga end with a translation of the sūtras of the *Śiva Svarodaya.* Since this text is already available in many publications, and since the 1967 edition of the *Svara Cintāmaṇi* can also be easily accessed, this book takes a different approach. I have decided to include in this publication my new translation of the seventh chapter of the *Svāccanda Tantra*, which deals directly with the Svara, and selected sections from the *Kālottara Tantra*, the two oldest extant descriptions of this teaching. To the best of my knowledge, this is the first time these chapters being presented in print in this way.

Moving Forward

Now that you understand where these teachings come from, you can read the rest of this book with a clearer sense of context. When I quote the *Śiva Svarodaya*, you'll know it's the foundational Hindu tantric text. When I reference the *Kālacakra Tantra*, you'll recognize it as the earlier Buddhist source. And when I offer my own interpretation, you'll understand that I'm continuing the tradition's long history of testing, questioning, and adapting ancient wisdom to new circumstances.

The texts mentioned above have preserved this knowledge across centuries. Now it's time to bring it alive in your own practice. You will do this by understanding the svara in your body, and specifically in your nose, which is the subject of our next chapter.

Chapter 4
All About the Nasal Cycle

It's All About the Nose

Have you ever noticed that one of your nostrils feels more open than the other, or that your sense of smell seems to fade mysteriously only to sharpen again a few moments later? This isn't something peculiar to you. It's part of a natural, biological rhythm we all share called the nasal cycle.

The nasal cycle is the unconscious, alternating partial congestion and decongestion of the nasal cavities that happens in humans as well as in some other mammals, such as cats and dogs. During a normal nasal cycle, one nostril becomes relatively more congested than the other, so that air flows predominantly through the less congested nostril, while the total resistance in the nose remains constant—meaning that the total amount of air passing through the nostrils stays about the same.

While this phenomenon has been recognized in many cultures for centuries, in the West the nasal cycle was first formally described by the German physician Richard Kaiser in 1895. The primary role of the nasal cycle is to support the healthy functioning of the nose, which in terms of respiration has three main jobs: warming the air from the external temperature to the body's internal temperature, humidifying the air, and filtering the air we breathe through the nose.

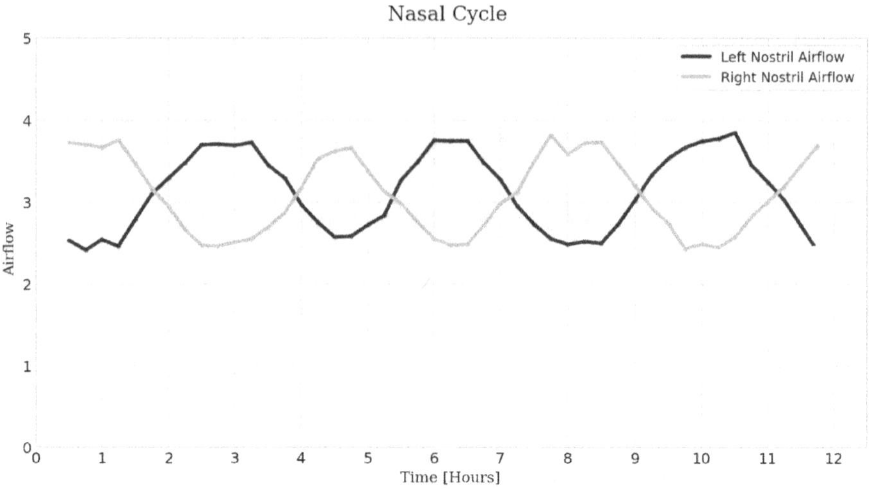

The humidifying and filtering functions of the nose depend on a layer of moist respiratory tissue inside the nasal cavity. Within this cavity, small hairs in the lining help filter foreign particles that arrive with the inhaled air, pushing these particles back outward and preventing them from entering the trachea and the rest of the respiratory system. In addition, the lining of the respiratory tract contains goblet cells that secrete mucus, which helps to moisten the air. As the air moves through the nose, it gradually dries this mucus. Once the mucus dries out, the air can no longer be moistened effectively, and the nasal hairs lose much of their ability to filter.

Rest, Recovery, and the Wisdom of Alternation

The presence of two independent nasal chambers (or foci) that function in an alternating pattern—one being more active than the other at any given moment—allows one side of the respiratory system to moisten itself while the other one is working and losing moisture to the air. Thus, while one nostril is active, the other is recuperating. The alternating pattern helps prevent excessive drying, crusting, and infection, which would likely develop in a static passage constantly exposed to airflow, especially in very dry environments such as deserts.

Another reason for the existence of this alternating nasal cycle lies in how it affects our olfaction, our sense of smell. At the heart of our sense of smell are specialized sensory receptors located in the olfactory epithelium, a small region inside the nasal cavity. These olfactory receptors interact chemically with specific odor molecules. When these volatile compounds come into contact with the receptors, they bind to them, triggering a biochemical process that eventually produces an electrical signal in the brain, which we experience as smell.

Once this chemical connection between the odor molecules and the receptors is formed, it takes time for it to be undone which is why smells seem to fade after a while. For instance, when you enter a perfume shop you are greeted by a cloud of scents—floral, musky, spicy, and more—and at first you can distinguish between them, but soon your brain filters them out. You then need a kind of reset, often achieved by smelling coffee, to regain your ability to differentiate between scents.

One of the functions of the alternating nasal cycle is to give our smell receptors a chance to reset, keeping the sense of smell clear and sensitive. It has also been found that each nostril perceives smells in slightly different ways. By naturally alternating the breath between one nostril and the other, the body creates a richer "smellscape" of the world around us, allowing a greater accuracy and clarity in how we perceive our environment.

Timing the Cycle

Modern medical research demonstrates that each cycle of breathing predominantly through one nostril and then shifting to the other can last anywhere from about 20 minutes to three and a half hours for a healthy individual, with an average of roughly two and a half hours for the entire cycle. In illness, this duration can stretch to four hours or more, showing considerable variability, whereas the traditional text *Śiva Svarodaya* mentions that the cycle should last exactly 60 minutes.

Most of the time, the nasal cycle runs quietly in the background, outside our conscious awareness. It usually becomes noticeable when we fall ill and one nostril becomes completely blocked. After 20 minutes, 60 minutes, or even several hours, the blockage may shift sides, making the alternation of the cycle easier to recognize.

From the perspective of Western science, the nasal cycle is driven by the autonomic nervous system, whose sympathetic and parasympathetic branches innervate the nasal cavity. The sympathetic branch is involved with activation, arousal, and activity, while the parasympathetic branch governs relaxation, rest, and rejuvenation. These two parts work in dynamic balance—when one becomes more active, the other quiets down.

When the sympathetic nerves in one nostril become active, the blood vessels in that nostril constrict, reducing the blood flow to the tissue. The tissue contracts and shrinks, increases the space in the nasal cavity for airflow effectively decongesting that nostril. After a while, sympathetic activity wanes and the parasympathetic nerves take over, increasing blood flow to the tissue, causing it to swell and narrow the passage, reducing airflow.

Four Medical Patterns of Nasal Cycling

Medical research describes four main nasal cycle patterns. The first, or classical pattern, is reciprocal congestion and decongestion with a constant total air volume—this is the regular nasal cycle, where breathing shifts from one nostril to another. The second is the parallel pattern, in which congestion or decongestion appears in both nasal cavities at the same time. The third is an irregular pattern, where nasal volume alternates without a defined pattern whereby the total volume may go up and down, and the nostrils may open and close without synchrony. Finally, the fourth is an acyclical pattern, in which the total nasal volume and the volume in each nostril do not differ, meaning there is effectively no nasal cycle at all.

While medical texts describe these four nasal patterns, this book follows a slightly different scheme of three or four breathing cycles. The first is breathing through the left nostril, also known as the *lunar svara*. The second is breathing through the right nostril, the *solar svara*. Together, these two form the classical nasal cycle. The third pattern, called *alternating fast*, partly overlaps with the medical "irregular" cycle: here, the breath shifts rapidly from left to right and back again within minutes or even within a single minute. However, in our tradition, that quick alternation is not seen as irregular, but as a rapid yet still orderly pattern. The final pattern is the *parallel svara*, corresponding to the medical description of parallel congestion or decongestion.

These four are the *svaras*, and it is by observing them—how they change, how they feel, and how the air flows through each nostril—that decisions and predictions are made in the science of Svara Yoga.

The nasal cycle isn't only about airflow. It also reflects deeper processes at work within us. To truly understand what the breath reveals, we must look beyond the physical body and into the subtle layers that ancient yogis mapped with astonishing precision. In the next chapter, we'll explore the structure of the human being according to yogic tradition, moving through the five kośas, the nāḍīs, and the vital force that flows through them: prāṇa.

Chapter 5
The Subtle Physiology of the Yogic Body

If breath is the bridge between body and mind, what exactly lies on either side of that bridge? The Indian science of *Svara Yoga* relies on the movement of certain, what we can call energies through certain channels, known as *nāḍīs*. In the coming chapters, I will explain the traditional Indian view of the structure of the human being—really, the human body or bodies—with the aim of clearing up any confusion you may have about this subtle anatomy.

The Five Kośas: Sheaths of Human Experience

In most yoga schools, we are taught a model in which the human being is composed of five bodies or five *kośas*, often translated as sheaths. The word sheath, like the sheath of a sword, suggests that each of these bodies that make up who we are is not who we truly are in our core; like a sword sheath, each one houses the inner consciousness, the self, the soul.

The usual list is as follows. The first body is the *Annamaya Kośa*, commonly called in English the physical body. *Anna* means food and *maya* means made of, so this is the sheath made of food, as the physical body is literally formed from food. The second body is the *Prāṇamaya Kośa*, the sheath made of *prāṇa*—the prāṇic body—sometimes called the energetic body, though more traditionally it can be understood as the body made of breath. The third body, *Manomaya Kośa*, is the sheath made of mind-stuff.

In the West this is often referred to as the emotional body or the astral body. The fourth body is the *Vijñānamaya Kośa*, the sheath made of *vijñāna*, or wisdom, and is normally called the wisdom body. Sometimes it's mistakenly labeled the mental body, but in truth the *Manomaya Kośa*—the third body—is the sheath of emotions and thoughts. The *Vijñānamaya Kośa* is not a mental body; it is a wisdom body, beyond the ordinary mind. Finally, the fifth body is *Ānandamaya Kośa*, the sheath made of *ānanda* or bliss.

This teaching about the five-layered structure of man comes from a very old text, the *Taittirīya Upaniṣad*, likely composed around the 5th century BCE. In the second chapter, the formation of the human being is explained:

From this very Self, *Ātman*, or pure consciousness, space came into being. From space, air. From air, fire. From fire, the waters. From the waters, the earth. From the earth, plants. From plants, food. And from food, man.

This is presented as the broad outline of how the universe was created and how the first body of man comes into being.

> "Now it will be described. A man here is formed from the essence of food. This here is his head, this is his right side, this is his left side, this is his torso, and this is the bottom on which he rests. Different from and lying within this man, formed from the essence of food, is the self consisting of life-breath, which suffuses that man completely. Now he has the appearance of man. So, corresponding to his manlike appearance, the self consisting of life-breath assumes a manlike appearance. Of this self, the head is simply the out-breath, the right side is the inter-breath, the left side is the in-breath, the torso is space and the bottom on which it rests is the earth.
>
> Next, it will describe the body made out of mind-stuff. Different from and lying within this self consisting of breath, is the self consisting of mind, which suffuses this other self completely.

Now he has the appearance of a man. So, corresponding to his manlike appearance, the self consisting of mind assumes a manlike appearance. Of this self, the head is simply the *yajus* formulas, the right side is the *ṛg* verses, the left side is the *sāman* chants, the torso is rules of substitution, and the bottom on which it rests is the *Atharva Āṅgiras.*

Next, the wisdom body will be described. Different from and lying within this self consisting of mind, is the self consisting of perception, which suffuses this other self completely. Now he has the appearance of man. So, corresponding to his manlike appearance, the self consisting of perception assumes a manlike appearance. Of this self, the head is simply faith, the right side is the truth, the left side is the real, the torso is the performance, and the bottom on which it rests is the celebration.

And finally, the *Ānandamaya Kośa* is described thus. Different from and lying within this self consisting of perception, is the self consisting of bliss, which suffuses this other self completely. Now he has the appearance of a man. So, corresponding to his manlike appearance, the self consisting of bliss assumes a manlike appearance. Of this self, the head is simply the pleasure, the right side is the delight, the left side is the thrill, the torso is the bliss, and the bottom on which it rests is Brahman".

Taittiriya Upanishad (2.1-5)

Annamaya Kośa

Let us look more closely at these five bodies in a way that is relevant to our subject. First is the physical body, the *Annamaya Kośa*, which is literally made of food and, from the traditional Indian perspective, is formed from the five gross elements of earth, water, fire, air, and space. Each of these elements represent a basic quality: solidity for earth, liquidity for water, movement and heat for fire, the gaseous state for air, and finally, space itself.

Prāṇamaya Kośa

The second body, *Prāṇamaya Kośa,* is the body made out of *prāṇa*. *Prāṇa* is that breath that enlivens the body. In the West, people sometimes call this the etheric body—Ether meaning something very rarefied— so this is seen as a body of very subtle and rarefied physical matter. It is also sometimes called the energetic body or the energetic double, but that language can be misleading, because people use the term *energy* to mean many different things. Some use it for subtle sensations that cannot be explained physically; others use it to describe the feeling that they get around a person— "this dude has a weird energy"—then they really mean the person is acting a little bit odd.

And so, I find it more helpful to use the traditional Indian term *prāṇa*. *Prāṇa* is that which enlivens the body. Sometimes *prāṇa* refers directly to the breath, but the word also has deeper meanings. This variety of meanings can create confusion, because different teachers in the Indian tradition use the word *prāṇa* at different times to denote different things. For some, *prāṇa* is just the breath coming in and out, and for others, it is a very deep function within the human being.

For our purposes here, the prāṇic body is the body made of breath, the body of vital, physical energy that animates the physical body.

The Indian tradition presents two views regarding the relationship between the pranic body and the physical body. According to one view the prāṇic body and the physical body are forever inseparable. The prāṇic body being always attached to the physical body and can in a sense, be considered a part of it. In this view they can never actually be separated; at death, the prāṇic body dissipates into space as the physical body that dissipates into nature. The second view is that the prāṇic body is separate from the physical body and is attached to the deeper sheaths, except for one of its components that are called *vāyus*.

The prāṇic body is comprised of, or governed by, ten *vāyus*, ten movements of *prāṇa*, usually described as five major *vāyus* and five secondary *vāyus*.

The five main *vāyus* are traditionally described as:

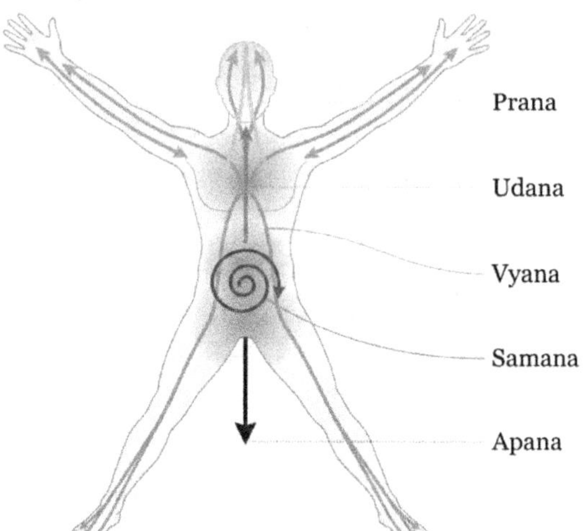

1. **Prāṇa Vāyu** – representing the movement of air inward and upward
2. **Apāna Vāyu** – representing the movement of air downward and outward.
3. **Udāna Vāyu** – having an upward movement and generating speech.
4. **Samāna Vāyu** – governing digestion & distribution.
5. **Vyāna Vāyu** – in charge of general maintenance of the body.

The five secondary *vāyus* fine-tune more specific functions:

6. **Nāga** – responsible for burping and hiccups.
7. **Kūrma** – in some texts, responsible for sneezing, and in others, for opening the eyes.
8. **Kṛkara** –sometimes linked with blinking, and sometimes with hunger and thirst.
9. **Devadatta** – responsible for yawning.
10. **Dhanañjaya** – associated either with twitching or with the decomposition of the body after death. This is the *vāyu* that never leaves the physical body, even in those traditions where the rest of the *prāṇic body may.*

Each prāṇa and sub-prāṇa is said to have a specific seat in the body . Prāṇa resides in the heart; Apāna in the region of the anus; *Samāna*, the digestive force, at the navel; *Udāna*, the upward-moving prāṇa, in the throat; and *Vyāna* is all-pervading, moving through the joints and all over the body.

Each one of the prāṇas is also associated with a different color: Prāṇa is like blood, red gem, or coral; *Apāna* has the color of the *indragopa* insect, with its white and red hues; *Samāna* has a tone between that of pure milk, crystal, or an oily and shining color—somewhere between *Prāṇa* and *Apāna*; *Udāna* is said to be pale white; and *Vyāna* is of the color of a ray of light, slightly yellowish.

Since ancient people observed that a living human being breathes, and that when the breath stops, the person died. It was therefore understood that the body which animates the physical body and carries the life force is this prāṇic body made of breath.

Manomaya Kośa, Vijñānamaya Kośa, Ānandamaya Kośa

Next is the *Manomaya Kośa*, the body made of emotions and thoughts. In Western esoteric language this is sometimes called the astral body. It is intimately linked—sometimes described as inseparable—from the *Vijñānamaya Kośa*, which is understood either as a the body of the deep subconscious and unconscious mind or as the body made of the very process of perception, akin to higher cognitive functioning. Finally comes the *Ānandamaya Kośa*, the sheath made out of bliss, though in some teachings this bliss is said to be shaped or conditioned by *karma*. This is the standard five-body scheme.

The Nāḍīs

Now we come to the *nāḍīs*. A *nāḍī* literally means a river or something that flows, and just as water flows through a river bed, prāṇa is said to flow through the *nāḍīs*. Alongside the *nāḍīs,* we have the *cakras*. Because prāṇa is described as flowing through the *nāḍīs*, many people assume that the *cakras* must be located in the prāṇic body, but the traditional view is a bit more complex and nuanced than that. To understand it, the five-body model needs to be set aside a moment in favor of another model that speaks of only three bodies.

It is important to remember that India preserved several parallel and sometimes competing theories and visions for explaining the human condition and the structure of the human being. The five-body *pañca-kośa* model that was just outlined is one such model, but it coexisted with parallel models such as the *trikāya* and the *śarīra-trayam*, both of which describe the human being as made of three parts.

The Kāya-Trayam Doctrine

In the kāya-trayam doctrine, the first part is called *sthūla śarīra*, the physical body. The second is the *sūkṣma śarīra,* the subtle body, which broadly corresponds to the combined *Prāṇamaya Kośa*, *Manomaya Kośa*, and *Vijñānamaya Kośa*. According to the *Tattva-bodha*, an Advaita Vedānta text originating from Ādi Śaṅkarācārya, this body is made up of seventeen components: the five sense organs, the five organs of action, the five prāṇas, the mind, and the intellect. Finally, the *kāraṇa śarīra,* the causal body (*kāraṇa* means cause), is the body that holds the karmic causes which create and underline all the other layers of our existence.

If the nāḍīs and cakras are placed within this three-body model, they belong to the subtle body. This means that when various texts describe the movement of prāṇa and the functioning of the cakras, they are talking about dynamics that happen in the interplay between the prāṇic body, the emotional-mental body, and the body of wisdom or perception. When it comes to the cakras, it is important to realize that throughout history there were multiple versions and models explaining them. The cakras are generally said to belong to the subtle body and are usually considered as deeper than the prāṇic layer alone; they are often aligned with the five elements along the central axis of the body. For the study of *Svara Yoga*, however, they are not very important.

The five-body model from the *Taittirīya Upaniṣad*, composed around the fifth century BCE, only entered the world of yoga much later, around the seventeenth century, through a text called *Yukta-Bhāvadeva*. By contrast, *Śiva Svarodaya*—the root text from which *Svara Yoga* evolved—comes from another stream altogether: the tantric tradition.

In the tantric view, the term prāṇa was also used, but not to refer to the layer closest to the physical body. Instead, the word prāṇa named that aspect of our being which is closest to Being itself. In this view, the physical body known as *deha* is the densest, most gross aspect of the human being. Next to it is *citta*, the mental or mind-heart body, equivalent to the *Manomaya Kośa*. Deeper than *citta* lies the *prāṇic body*, the body made of prāṇa. In the tradition from which this teaching comes, prāṇa is not merely a life force—it is the power that moves both mind and body.

Beyond *prāṇa* we find *śūnya*, emptiness, and finally beyond *śūnya* is *cit,* consciousness itself. When we understand that the writer of our main text had this as his underlying model of the universe; when we understand that in his conception the layer in which prāṇa flowed was closer to what the Vedāntins call the causal body—the *Ānandamaya Kośa* or the *liṅga śarīra*, it becomes clear why the flow of prāṇa through the nāḍīs was believed to determine one's karma, and shape one's destiny.

For the writer of the *Śiva Svarodaya* and for those yogis who practiced *Svara Yoga*, *svara*—the breath—was never just the air moving in and out of the body. It was the movement of prāṇa through the nāḍīs, in the deepest recesses of the human being. And this prāṇa, understood not only as the life force but as the very power that drives the entire universe, when passing through the different nāḍīs, changed everything about the world around it. How this prāṇa governs human consciousness and destiny is the focus of our next chapter.

Chapter 6
The 3 Nadis and Their Correlation to the Svaras

The concept of subtle structures through which *prāṇa* flows is extremely ancient. The word *nāḍī* comes from the root *nad* or *nāda*, which either means "to flow" or refers to something hollow through which other things can move. In the Indian tradition, it is said that there are 72,000 *nāḍīs*, as stated in the *Bṛhadāraṇyaka Upaniṣad*. Or, in other sources, such as the *Prapañcasāra Tantra* or the *Śiva Saṃhitā,* this number expands to 300,000 or even 350,000 *nāḍīs*. The names of these texts are stated here so that you can question and verify what is said, rather than taking this information at face value.

These *nāḍīs* are said to permeate the entire body. Some texts claim that the *nāḍīs* originate from the heart. Some suggest that the *nāḍīs* originate from a point just below the navel known as *kaṇḍa*, "theegg", which practitioners of *qìgōng* would recognize as corresponding to the lower *Dāntián*. Within these *nāḍīs,* the various forms of *prāṇa* move as *vāyus*, or winds; the five main *vāyus* and the five secondary *vāyus* together support different functions throughout the body.

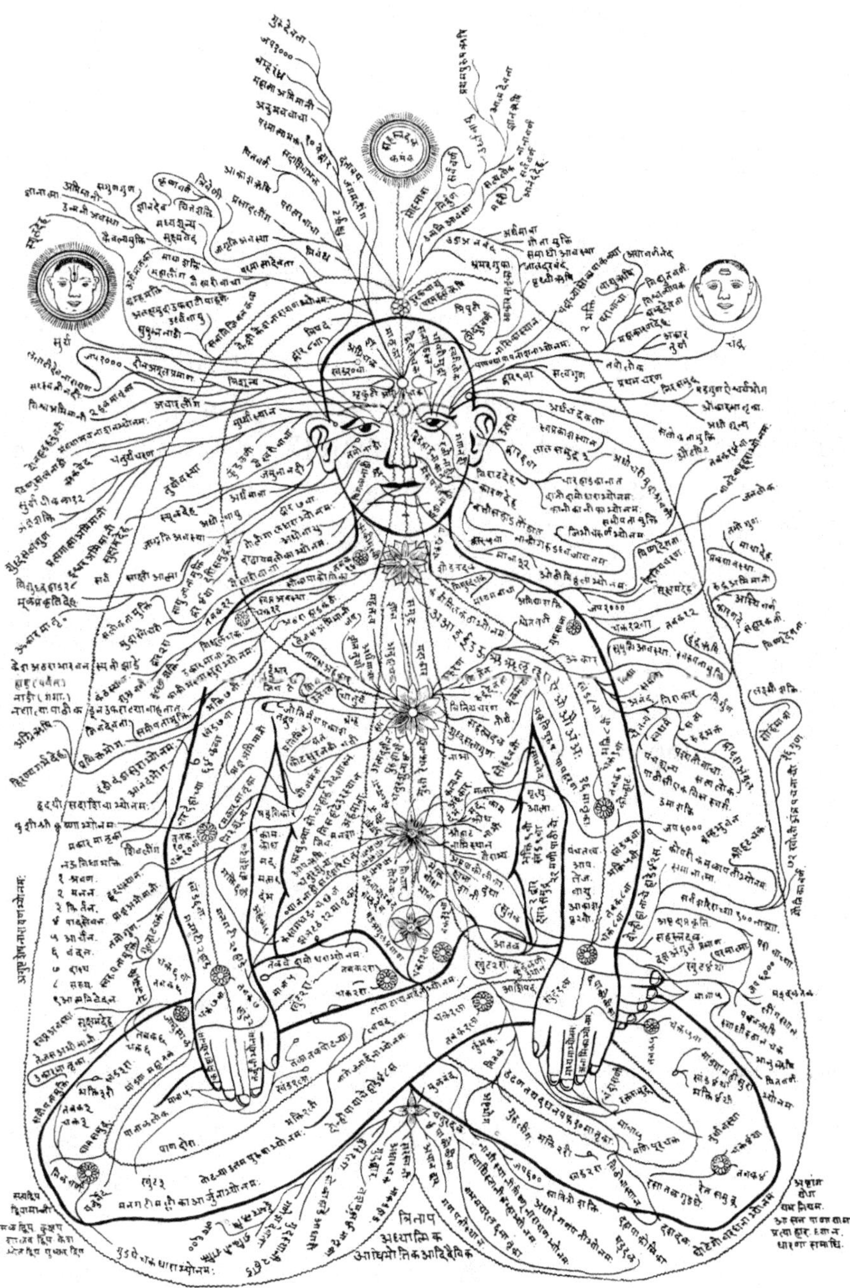

Now, out of the 72,000 (or, in some accounts, 350,000) *nāḍīs*, most texts single out "a hundred and something" as particularly important — often

101, 111, or 114. From these, usually 10 or 11 are highlighted and named. The *Śiva Svarodaya*, the main text to teach *Svara Yoga*, describes ten major *nāḍīs* that connect the center of the being to the ten doorways of the body: **Gāndhārī**, which connects to the left eye; **Hastijihvā**, to the right eye; **Pūṣā**, to the right ear; **Yaśasvinī**, to the left ear; **Alambuṣā**, to the mouth; **Kuhu**, to the reproductive organs; **Śaṅkhinī**, to the rectum; **Iḍā**, to the left nostril; **Piṅgalā**, to the right nostril; and **Suṣumṇā**, to the *brahmarandhra,* the fontanelle at the crown of the head. In adults, the *brahmarandhra* no longer an actual opening but the location where the bones of the skull meet; in babies, this spot is open and gradually closes over time in the first months of life, forming the cranial sutures. In yoga, this point is regarded as a subtle opening that can be "re-opened" later in life, allowing access to higher states of consciousness. Out of these ten *nāḍīs*, the three most important are the **Iḍā**, **Piṅgalā**, and **Suṣumṇā**. In fact, in the most ancient references to the *nāḍīs,* only these three are mentioned explicitly; the others appear later in the tradition, at least in name.

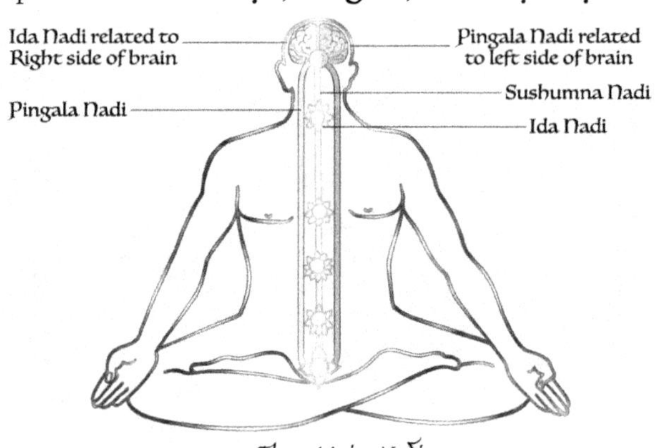

Three Major Nadis

The Suṣumṇā Nāḍī

The *Suṣumṇā nāḍī* is described as the central channel of the subtle body. In some traditions, it is stated to run exactly through the middle of the body: if you draw a line from the perineum to the crown of the head straight through the center —not along the spine—that line represents the *Suṣumṇā*, or the central channel. This view is especially common in Tibetan yogas and tantras. In other teachings, the *Suṣumṇā* is described as running along the spine itself and is considered to be the subtle aspect, the subtle correlate to the spinal cord. Indeed, just as the spinal cord connects the brain (the higher functions) with the rest of the body, in subtle anatomy the *Suṣumṇā* is the channel along which the *cakras* are strung and is considered the spiritual axis of the being.

On either side of the *Suṣumṇā* lie the *Iḍā nāḍī* on the left and the *Piṅgalā nāḍī* on the right. They are said to run about an inch to either side of the spine, arising from the *Mūlādhāra* (sometimes identified with the gonads) and ascend up to the third eye or to their respective nostrils. In some descriptions, *Iḍā* always stays to the left of the spine and *Piṅgalā* to the right; in others, the *nāḍīs* crisscross each other, intersecting at each point where a *cakra* is said to lie along the *Suṣumṇā*. This crossing over one another creates the well-known image of the caduceus: a central staff with two serpents weaving back and forth along its length.

Iḍā: The Lunar Channel

The Sanskrit word *iḍā* can be translated as "comfort", so *Iḍā nāḍī* is the comfortable *nāḍī*, and when prāṇa flows through the *Iḍā* we become comfortable and there is a natural tendency to turn toward relaxation and restfulness. The *Śiva Svarodaya* likens the nature of the Iḍā to the energy of the moon: Iin the Indian view, the sun is considered hot and burning, and indeed, in many contexts it is considered a negative force, while the moon's light is the cooling, calming, and nourishing. The moon is said to bring moisture and humidity to the world and is linked to the water element, while the sun dries out the earth. For this reason, Iḍā nāḍī is known as the *Candra-nāḍī —Candra* being the name of the moon in the Indian tradition—or the lunar nāḍī, with a cooling, relaxing, and introverting quality.

Iḍā is said to arise on the left side of the *Mūlādhāra cakra* at the root of the spine, or sometimes from the left gonad. Ascending along the spine—either staying consistently on the left or crisscrossing back and forth—it reaches the left nostril and connects to the left side of the Ājñā cakra (the third eye). The Śiva Svarodaya teaches that the left nāḍī is active and activated when we breathe in and out through the left nostril, and that the energy passing through the Iḍā nāḍī is manas-śakti, the energy of mind, so all mental activity is said to function through the action of this channel. The Iḍā is depicted as white in color, associated with the moon and with tamas, one of the three guṇas, or fundamental karmic tendencies of nature, an association that is central to how the flow of *prāṇa* in these three *nāḍīs* is understood to influence not only our behavior and tendencies but also our *karma* and therefore our destiny.

Piṅgalā: The Solar Channel

Piṅgalā means "tawny" or reddish-brown and refers to the reddish-brown prāṇic channel on the right side of the body. It is also called Sūrya-nāḍī, the solar channel, with *Sūrya* being the Sun god in the Indian tradition. Piṅgalā carries the *prāṇa* of the sun, it is considered to be heating and is connected to the the *guṇa* of rajas.

It's also mentioned that while the energy of the mind flows through the Candra-nāḍī, the Piṅgalā nāḍī carries prāṇa-śakti.

The Piṅgalā is said to emerge from the right side of the *Mūlādhāra cakra* (or from the right gonad) and to travel upward either parallel to the spine toward the right nostril—with an offshoot linking into the right side of the third eye, or, in some descriptions, touching the spine and intersecting with the Iḍā nāḍī, or even crossing back and forth depending on the text.

From personal experience with meditation and *prāṇāyāma*, meditating on Iḍā as always residing on the left and connected to the left side of the body, and Piṅgalā always residing on and connected to the right reveals a clear pattern: when attention is placed on the left nāḍī, sensations and imagery related to the left side of the body become more vivid, and when working on the right nāḍī, the right side becomes more prominent. From such experimentations I have come to the conclusion that Iḍā consistently remains on the left and Piṅgalā on the right, though you are encouraged to try this directly and notice what arises for you.

Suṣumṇā: The Central Channel

Finally, at the center of the body—or along the spine—lies the *Suṣumṇā nāḍī*. *Suṣumṇā* can be translated as "supremely gracious" or "compassionate", and is known as the channel through which *Kuṇḍalinī* passes, determining our level of consciousness. This is the axis mundi of the body: all of the *cakras* sprout from it, and in some visions all 72,000 *nāḍīs* arise from the Iḍā and Piṅgalā, which themselves spring from the Suṣumṇā *nāḍī*.

If this is taken metaphorically, the experience of yoga—union or oneness—arises from the experience of the Suṣumṇā *nāḍī*, where all of our *prāṇas*, all of our energies, are gathered and unified, creating a state of consciousness of oneness. When we enter into duality, this unified consciousness is said to split into two currents—the Iḍā and the Piṅgalā—and from these two archetypal poles of plus and minus, sun and moon, the other 72,000 branch out, much as the body differentiates around the neural tube, the central channel around which our entire symetrical body is developed during fetal growth.

Suṣumṇā is said to be of the element of fire and consciousness itself. It is described as being of of all three *guṇas—rajas*, *tamas*, and *sattva*. The Suṣumṇā is described as having three layers. The external layer is called *Suṣumṇā*; within it runs *Citrinī*, as fine as a spider's thread and threaded through all of the *cakras*; at the very core is *Brahma-nāḍī*, the innermost layer of the Suṣumṇā that extends to the *brahmarandhra*, the opening of Brahmā at the crown that opens to the cosmos. This innermost channel is of the nature of pure consciousness and bliss, and many yogic techniques aim specifically to enter and awaken this most subtle aspect of Suṣumṇā.

Some texts offer slightly different names for these inner channels. For example, in the *Lalitā-Sahasranāma*, the fiery red Suṣumṇā has within it a *Vajra-nāḍī* of a solar nature and a pale, nectar-dropping *Citrinī-nāḍī* of a lunar nature—like inner forms of Piṅgalā and Iḍā manifesting themselves inside Suṣumṇā. The moon-natured Citrinī-nāḍī is said to be responsible for visions and altered states of consciousness, revealing something about how the Iḍā and Piṅgalā manifest within the central channel. It is within the Suṣumṇā *nāḍī* that Kuṇḍalinī rises to create these altered states of consciousness.

A Note on Yin and Yang

When exploring Iḍā and Piṅgalā, another familiar pair often comes to mind: *Yin* and *Yang*. The concept of Yin and Yang originate in Chinese philosophy as opposite but interconnected forces. The original term simply meant the sunny and shaded sides of the hill, but this later became a metaphor for the light and dark aspects of the *Dao*, the unifying principle in Chinese mysticism. In this cosmology, the material energy of the universe is called *Qi*, and Qi operates in two complementary ways—Yin and Yang. In fact, according to this, any division into two will align with Yin and Yang. Thus Yin (dark/black) and Yang (light/white) may also be equated with water (Yin) and fire (Yang), expansion (Yin) and contraction (Yang), and so on. Even "good" and "bad" as moral categories can be mapped onto Yin and Yang, though that association stems more from Confucian influence than from the original Daoist teaching.

Classical Chinese philosophers described Yin as the lunar, cooling aspect connected with darkness, passivity, negativity, destruction, nighttime, receptivity, the earth, and femininity. Yin was characterized as slow, soft, yielding, diffuse, cold, wet, and passive. Yang, in contrast, is the light or sunny side of life: open, overt, belonging to the world—described as fast, hard, solid, focused, hot or warm, dry, and active. Yang is linked with fire, sky and air, the sun, positivity, creation, daytime, and masculinity.

Everything in nature is seen as a blend of these two—Yin and Yang. Thus A concentrated seed is Yang, while sprouting, the release and expansion of this concentrated form, is a Yin process; winters, being cold, are Yin, while summers, being hot, are Yang. Foods, behaviors, concepts, thoughts, and ideas can all be defined as more Yin or more Yang. And of course, this mapping is also projected onto human beings, whereby femininity is classified as Yin and masculinity as Yang.

Before continuing, it is worth acknowledging today's cultural discussions about the meanings of "masculinity" and "femininity", and about the distinctions between "male" and "female". Male and female are often defined biologically, especially in terms of chromosomal makeup, though even here other factors may come into play. Masculine and feminine, meanwhile, are seen by some as based on biology while others hold they are cultural constructs. This important conversation is beyond the scope of this book; what is being described here simply reflects what traditional sources say. Whether these ideas feel accurate or useful is for you to decide.

Returning to our main thread, Yin was taken to incorporate everything considered feminine and Yang everything considered masculine. Over time, this framework was applied to the Iḍā and Piṅgalā, where Iḍā became "the feminine *nāḍī*", and Piṅgalā "the masculine *nāḍī*". Since Yin and Yang were seen to cover the whole of existence by dividing it into two fundamental aspects, the Iḍā and Piṅgalā *nāḍīs* came to represent the same polarity within yogic circles. Iḍā was therefore linked with actions considered feminine—receptive, gentle, nourishing, calming, restoring, creative.—while the Piṅgalā *nāḍī* was everything considered masculine—spatial, aggressive, analytical, active, outgoing, arousing. While this cross-cultural mapping may hold some truth, it is important to remember that this is a relatively recent development, rather than an original feature of the classical yogic tradition.

Thus, our three *nāḍīs* can be seen together: Iḍā, considered the feminine channel; Piṅgalā, considered the masculine channel; and Suṣumṇā, considered the neuter—the balanced, undivided channel residing in the middle. These three are also related to the three *guṇas*, the universal qualities that shape and govern our destiny, which will be explored in the next chapter.

Chapter 7
The Three Guṇas and Their Role in Svara Yoga

Let us now look more deeply at the three guṇas and how they relate to *Svara Yoga*. In yogic philosophy, the entire material universe emanates from a foundational substrate known as *prakṛti*, while at the same time the world is said to emanate from consciousness itself. Consciousness, the being, the soul, is termed *puruṣa*, and it exists together with *prakṛti*.

Prakṛti literally means "nature", but in its original sense it refers to pure potential, not to anything already manifest. Within *prakṛti* reside three primary guṇas, or qualities of energy, which give rise to the fundamental aspects of all of existence: energy, matter, and consciousness itself.

These three guṇas are *tamas*, associated with darkness and chaos; *rajas*, linked with activity and passion; and *sattva*, which represents beingness and harmony. They can be understood as three fundamental forces governing both creation and consciousness. In this sense, they are karmic, or causal, energies—*kāraṇa*-śaktis—that cause everything else to unfold.

Tamas is the energy that lulls consciousness to sleep. It is the force that generates the world and makes consciousness lose itself within that world. *Rajas* is the force that drives consciousness into action, animating it to live, move, and engage with the world. *Sattva*, finally, is the quality that awakens consciousness and turns away from the world—from *māyā*, illusion—toward the recognition of its own true nature, its beingness.

Within prakṛti, these three guṇas exist in a state of utter equilibrium. As long as they are fully balanced, existence does not unfold. At a certain point, however, this equilibrium is shaken, and through that disturbance the universe is created.

What Is a Guṇa?

In yoga and Ayurveda, the Sanskrit word *guṇa* denotes a quality, , attribute, or tendency that exists in every single thing. The three guṇas—*tamas*, *rajas*, and *sattva*—simultaneously permeate all beings and objects, albeit in varying proportions.

The guṇas are in constant flux; they are constantly shifting in a playful dance called *māyā*, the grand illusion we experience as the world. Their ongoing interplay shapes the core attributes of individuals and things, and profoundly influences the trajectory and evolution of each life, according to each individual's unique mix of the three.

Human beings have a special capacity: they can consciously influence the relative strength of these guṇas in their bodies and minds. While the guṇas cannot be removed, they can be purposefully influenced through choices in action, lifestyle, and thought. For yogic practitioners, understanding the guṇas becomes an inner compass, helping to guide decisions toward greater balance, clarity, and harmony.

Defining the Three Guṇas

Tamas embodies darkness, inertia, inactivity, and materiality. It arises from ignorance, veiling spiritual truth and leading beings to become lost in *māyā*. *Tamas* is not inherently negative—it give solidarity to the world and enables sleep—but when it exists in excess, it may show up as laziness, disgust, attachment, depression, helplessness, doubt, guilt, shame, boredom, addiction, hurt, sadness, apathy, confusion, grief, dependency, or ignorance.

Rajas represents energy, action, change, and movement. It manifests as attraction, longing, and attachment, binding us to the fruits of our actions and keeping us engaged and busy in the world. When excessive, *rajas* can manifest as anger, euphoria, anxiety, fear, irritation, worry, restlessness, stress, courage, rumination, fierce determination, and even chaos. Despite its instability, *rajas* plays an essential role in spiritual life by agitating tamas and catalyzing awakening and transformation.

Sattva is the quality of harmony, balance, joy, and intelligence. It brings about delight, happiness, peace, health, freedom, love, compassion, equanimity, empathy, friendliness, focus, self-control, satisfaction, trust, fulfillment, calm, bliss, cheerfulness, gratitude, fearlessness, and selflessness. Yogis consciously aim to cultivate *sattva,* because it gently weakens both *rajas* and *tamas* and supports the path toward liberation.

Working With the Guṇas

Each guṇa can be amplified or diminished through diet, lifestyle, and thought.

To reduce *tamas,* it is recommended to avoid tamasic foods such as alcohol, drugs, tobacco, red meat, spoiled or rotten food, items high in artificial additives like sweeteners and preservatives, greasy or heavy meals, stale or leftover dishes, highly processed or refined foods, garlic, raw onions, mushrooms, and other fungal or mycelial substances. Fermented foods created by fungal decomposition—such as many moldy cheeses—are considered tamasic, while those produced by bacterial fermentation, like yogurt, are not. Behaviors that increase tamas include oversleeping, overeating, chronic inactivity, passivity, and prolonged exposure to fear-based situations.

To reduce *rajas*, it is advised to avoid overly spicy foods, fried items, dishes with excessive salt or sugar, coffee and energy drinks, and highly stimulating meals—such as those with many ingredients, complex or intense spices, or extreme temperatures. Foods from the nightshade family (like aubergine), hard-to-digest beans, and deep-fried items should be minimized. At a lifestyle level, reducing *rajas* means avoiding over-exercising and overworking, limiting loud or chaotic environments (such as constant loud music), calming excessive thinking or consumption, speaking less, listening more, and practicing mindfulness. It also helps to avoid extended exposure to strong sunlight and favoring cooler, softer light. In work, the ideal is to practice *karma yoga*—offering your efforts for the benefit of others, without attachment to the outcome.

At the same time, in situations of excess *tamas*, it may be helpful to increase rajas in order to ignite energy and break through inertia. If you are feeling depressed, procrastinating, fearful, or stuck in avoidance, consciously cultivating rajas can catalyze movement and change.

To increase *sattva*, one is encouraged to eat foods like raw nuts and seeds, pure oils, sweet and mild fruits (while avoiding very sour or pungent ones), mild vegetables, whole grains, easily digestible lentils, and natural sweeteners such as honey. Herbs like tulsi (holy basil) are also beneficial. Dairy products may be sattvic if acquired ethically—for example, in certain Indian āśrams, cows are milked only after giving birth naturally, only after the calf has fed fully, and are cared for with deep love and respect. In contrast, industrial dairy production common in the West is seen as tamasic due to the suffering it involves. Ultimately, sattvic food is that which is grown, prepared, and eaten with mindfulness, gratitude, and love—from the planting of the seed until the food reaches the mouth.

Beyond diet, *sattva* is nourished by a joyous and simple life, time in nature, positive thinking, regular yoga and meditation, and living in accordance with the *yamas* and *niyamas*, the ethical codes of yoga.

Transcending the Guṇas

Of the three guṇas, *sattva* is the most supportive for spiritual life. Yet all three guṇas, including *sattva,* are said to create attachment and thus bind the self to the ego. As the *Bhagavad Gītā* teaches:

"When one rises above the three guṇas that originate in the body, one is freed from birth, old age, disease, and death, and attains enlightenment".

For the yogi who seeks final liberation, the path is to first cultivate *sattva* and then ultimately transcend all three guṇas entirely.

The Guṇas and the Nāḍīs

Svara Yoga is not merely a philosophy of transcendence; it is a practical science for living in the world. Within this perspective, the Iḍā nāḍī, or left channel, is connected with *tamas*—the energy of manifestation. The Piṅgalā nāḍī, or right channel, is associated with *rajas*, and the Suṣumṇā nāḍī, the central channel, is connected primarily with *sattva* as well as with the harmonious balance of all three guṇas, since it consists of three internal *nāḍīs* layered within one another.

At the deepest level, the three guṇas are seen as root karmic forces that shape the overall trajectory of our lives. Since they reside at the very base of our being, they guide our actions and their results—our karma. If the guṇas can be influenced through lifestyle, behavior, and diet, then our karma, too, can be gently altered.

Moreover, since the guṇas are linked to the left and right nostrils, *Svara Yoga* teaches that by manipulating the breath—by breathing through the left or right nostril—we can attune to specific karmic energies and steer our destiny. This is the very heart of *Svara Yoga*. By noticing which *nāḍī* is active at any given moment and choosing actions that match that current, we can move in harmony with the prevailing energetic current. If the timing is wrong, the instruction is simple: wait for the breath—*svara*—to change. This alignment of timing, breath, and action is what gives *Svara Yoga* its seemingly magical quality. The idea is that karma comes into alignment when what you do and how you breathe are in harmony, and through this alignment, destiny can begin to align.

Historically, this is why the teachings of *Svara Yoga* were treated as secret. It was believed that by knowing which karmic energies—*rajas*, *tamas*, or *sattva*— were flowing at a given moment, practitioners could influence events that seemed far beyond the reach of personal control.

Imagine: simply by observing which *svara* is dominant at a given moment and adjusting your actions accordingly, you could change the outcome of your life. And if the moment isn't right? You do nothing. You wait until it is. This is the spiritual explanation of how *Svara Yoga* works.

Before turning to the scientific understanding of *Svara Yoga*, the next step is to learn how to observe the nasal cycle, recognize which *svara* is active, and align your activities accordingly. What guidance does the *Śiva Svarodaya* offer for times when the Lunar Svara (left nostril) is dominant? What is recommended when the Solar Svara (right nostril) is flowing? These questions form the foundation of the practical application of *Svara Yoga*.

PART II:
THE PRACTICE OF SVARA YOGA

Chapter 8
How to Identify the Active Svara

Before we can do any work with the svara, it is essential to be able to recognize which svara is active. In this chapter I will guide you step by step through traditional and modern methods for identifying which nostril—and therefore which *svara*—is active at any given moment.

Preparing to Sense the Svara

Find a comfortable sitting position and, if you wish, close your eyes to help you turn inward. Closing the eyes is not strictly necessary to check your *svara*, but it can heighten awareness of the subtle bodily sensations that will guide this exploration.

Begin by observing your natural breath. Without changing anything, simply notice:

- Can you feel the air moving more freely through one nostril?
- Is there a slight dominance in airflow on one side?

If you cannot tell yet, try this:

1. **Breathe consciously through both nostrils.**
   Inhale and exhale with just a bit more effort than usual.

2. **Observe the sensation.**
   Does the air move more smoothly through one nostril than the other?

Now, gently close one nostril—it doesn't matter which—and inhale and exhale through the open nostril. Notice how much effort it takes, or how easy it feels, then switch sides and repeat.

Can you sense which nostril is more open and which is more closed? Once you have identified this, breathe again through both nostrils together and see whether you can now feel that subtle imbalance even with both open. Becoming familiar with this delicate perception is the foundation of *Svara Yoga* practice.

Method 1: The Palm Test

Place your left hand just beneath your nostrils, about 2–3 cm away, level with your mouth. The back of your palm should face upward toward the nose. Exhale gently through both nostrils and notice where you feel the gust of air more strongly—closer to your fingertips or nearer your wrist.

- If the air is felt closer to the fingertips while using the left hand, it means that your right nostril (the solar *svara*) is active.
- If the sensation is stronger closer to the wrist, your left nostril (the lunar *svara*) is dominant.

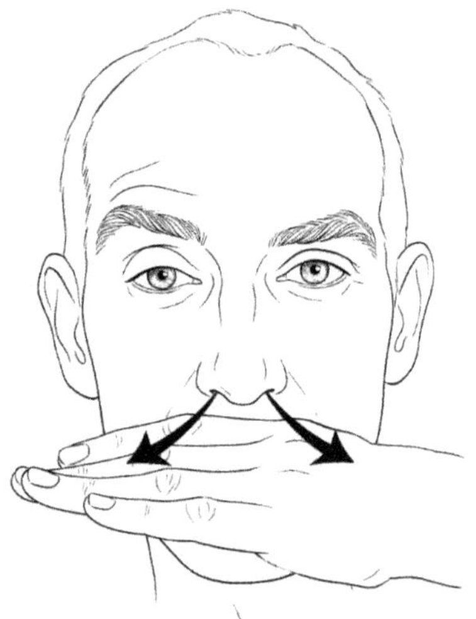

You can enhance the sensitivity of this method by slightly moistening the back of your hand—traditionally, yogis simply lick the hand, though you may also use a little water. Then exhale again and observe not only the gust of air but also the cooling sensation created as the moisture evaporates. Where is the sensation most distinct—near the fingers or near the wrist?

If your fingertips and wrist have different levels of sensitivity, experiment by placing your hand a bit farther down the forearm. Often, the tiny hairs on the forearm will register the movement of air more clearly, making it easier to sense which side is more active.

Method 2: The Mirror or Smartphone Test

Traditionally, yogis used a mirror to determine which nostril was dominant. You can do the same today with a mirror, a smartphone screen, or any glossy surface. Hold it just below your nose, where it touches the upper lip, and exhale gently through both nostrils. Immediately lift the phone or mirror and look at the condensation marks that appear.

- If the mark is longer or denser on the right side, the right nostril is dominant.
- If the mark is larger on the left side, the left nostril is dominant.

Repeat this process if needed. The condensation pattern does more than identify the active *svara*; it also hints at how the five elements are operating within each *svara* at that moment. The *Tantras* describe subtle variations in these shapes as indicators of which types of actions are auspicious at different times.

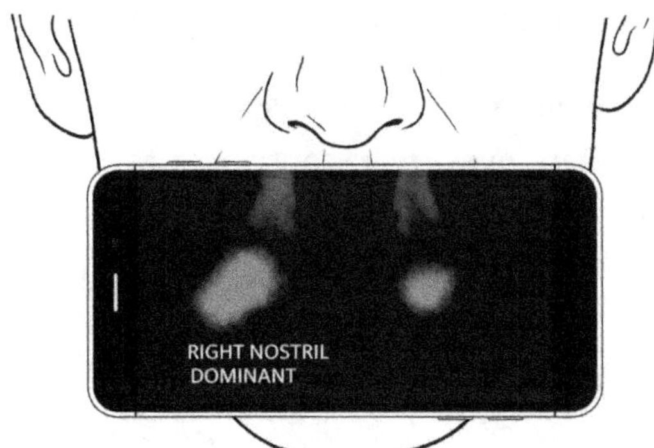

A Note on Septal Deviation

Modern anatomy adds an important nuance to this work. Some people have a deviated nasal septum—a slight or significant bend in the thin wall dividing the nostrils—which can make one side seem permanently more open, regardless of the svara's actual alternation.

The septum itself is a bony and cartilaginous wall that divides the left and right nasal passages, covered by a mucous membrane that keeps the nasal passages moist and protected. When it is properly aligned, it allows balanced airflow through both sides, supporting healthy breathing and clear vocal resonance.

When the septum is deviated, it can lead to chronic congestion, poor sinus drainage, snoring, or even sleep apnea, and can sometimes contribute to headaches or facial pain. Beyond these physical effects, continual dominance of one nostril can disrupt the balance of the nervous system:

- **Left-dominant breathing** (lunar, Iḍā) keeps the body in a parasympathetic "rest and digest" mode, and if it's chronically dominant, it may lead to fatigue, lethargy, or mild depression.
- **Right-dominant breathing** (solar, Piṅgalā) activates the sympathetic "fight or flight" response. Long-term dominance on this side may manifest as agitation, anxiety, or even panic attacks.

While left-side dominance is usually less problematic, persistent right-nostril dominance can, over time, contribute to hormonal imbalances and may even trigger chronic migraines.

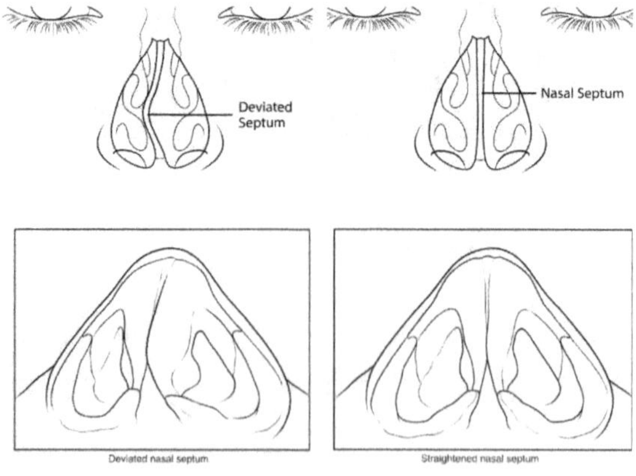

The Svara and Migraine Relief

As you may know, I am a somatic therapist, and actually have developed my own method for alleviating headaches and even migraine attacks. Although this method deserves—and will eventually be presented in—its own book, a simple technique that draws directly from *Svara Yoga* principles can be shared here.

When a migraine attack first begins, it can often be alleviated by activating the left nostril: lie on the right side so the left nostril is uppermost, or gently close the right nostril and breathe only through the left.

This shifts the body into parasympathetic activation, calming the system and often stopping the attack if caught early enough. This technique is most effective at the onset of symptoms, before the full cascade of a migraine has unfolded.

Causes and Remedies for Septal Deviation

There are several possible causes of septal deviation:

- **Congenital factors** - present from birth due to developmental irregularities.
- **Aging** - gradual shifting of the septum over time.
- **Environmental influences** - including chronic irritation or inflammation of the nasal tissues.
- **Trauma** - injury to the nose or head.

Around 30% of people are born with some degree of deviation, usually mild, and most only become aware of it when they begin a subtle practice like *Svara Yoga*.

Treatment options vary. Medications such as decongestants or corticosteroid nasal sprays can ease symptoms but do not change the underlying structure. Yogic nasal cleansing, or *jala neti*, can help clear blockages and improve airflow, while nasal dilators—external or internal—may mechanically widen the passages. Surgery (septoplasty) is generally reserved for more severe cases, such as significant sleep apnea or pronounced asymmetry.

I generally recommend avoiding surgery unless clearly necessary: a mild deviation is usually manageable and even educational, highlighting just how sensitive and dynamic the nasal cycle truly is. In some rare cases, however, particularly when chronic depression or hormonal imbalance appears related to a severe deviation, surgery can be genuinely life-changing.

Working with Septal Deviation in Svara Yoga

To determine whether you have a septal deviation, you can use the mirror test described earlier. Notice not only which nostril is active, but also whether the shape of condensation remains consistently larger on one side, even as the *svara* alternates.

You can also test over time—every 30, 60, or 90 minutes. Under usual circumstances, the active nostril alternates. If it doesn't, or if one side always appears physically wider even when inactive, you likely have a septal deviation.

In most cases, this simple awareness is enough. There is no need to "fix" the deviation unless it creates significant symptoms. However, if you do begin to notice life patterns that mirror chronic dominance of one nostril—such as anxiety with right-side dominance or lethargy with left-side dominance—you can start using *Svara Yoga* intentionally to restore balance.

Now that you know how to identify whether the lunar (left) or solar (right) svara is active, you are ready to explore how to choose actions aligned with each svara in order to achieve success.

Chapter 9
What Should You Do on Each of the Svaras

We now arrive at one of the core teachings of Svara Yoga: the actions which are recommended— and those best avoided —when each svara is active. Remember that the idea behind Svara Yoga is that both human beings and nature undergo certain cycles, and when we align our actions with these cycles, we are promised to receive the maximum return on our efforts.

Now that you know how to determine which svara is active, we can explore which actions are recommended to be done when your lunar svara is active, which are appropriate when your solar svara is active, and which are suited to the middle, the Suṣumṇā Svara, when neither lunar nor solar is primary.

The guidance on what to do and what to avoid is strewn throughout *Śiva Svarodaya* —there is one main section dedicated for each svara, but many additional hints are floating across the text.

I have gathered all these scattered instructions into a single accessible list. Most of this list is drawn from the *Śiva Svarodaya*, with additions from the *Svara Cintāmaṇi*, as well as from texts such as the *Kālacakra Tantra*, which, as I mentioned earlier, likely served as the basis for this teaching.

As you read this list I suggest to meditate on the information and try to see if you can discover a common ground or shared logic between the various pieces of advice. Some items may seem quite random, so consider this an invitation to look for the deeper connections linking them all.

The list will follow the order given in the *Śiva Svarodaya* rather than any new system of organization, so it will not be arranged in a strict hierarchy or scheme. At times, there may be some repetitions when similar information appears in different sources.

The Lunar Svara (Left Svara / Iḍā Nāḍī)

Here is the list of actions that Svara Yoga recommends when our left Svara is active.

Starting a short journey (longer journeys, are reserved for the right svara); travel toward the west or south; beginning a journey with the left leg; lightly touch the left side of your face in the morning; take an even number of steps when setting out; Leaving the house, digging small or large wells and ponds, consecrating a deity's idol, arranging marriages, offering donations, and making journeys are all favorable.

This svara is also recommended for acquiring clothes, ornaments, and decorative articles; purchasing jewelry, undertaking stable or long-term actions; constructing an *āśram* or temple; collecting things,; and doing peaceful work. It supports obtaining nourishment, taking divine medicines and chemicals, meeting one's spiritual master, making friends, collecting, engaging in commercial business, collecting grain, and entering a new house. Sowing seeds, offering service, performing auspicious works, forming alliances, preparing to go outside, and meeting friends and relatives are likewise advised, as are activities connected to birth and death and the performing of religious rites.

When the lunar svara flows, it is a good time for taking initiation and practicing one's mantra, beginning studies, bringing cattle home, and treating otherwise incurable diseases. It is recommended for addressing one's master, reading sūtras concerning the science of time — past, present, and future—keeping a horse or elephants in the stable, mounting a horse or elephant, practicing archery, keeping and securing wealth, performing charity, and serving others. Dancing and studying dance, entering a city or village, applying tilak (the mark Indians traditionally wear on the forehead), acquiring land, playing music, singing, and interacting with relatives are all considered auspicious

In addition, the lunar svara is favorable for collecting firewood, helping those in acute sufferings—such as people with fever or in an unconscious state—for welcoming the arrival of rain, and for counteracting poison. It is recommended for worshiping the spiritual teacher, applying dental decorations for women, drinking water, urinating, and getting out of bed. Calm and silent work, especially that which requires mental activity, is well supported, as are charitable actions, approaching those in senior positions, sowing seeds, taking a hot bath, and anointing the body with oil.

Food Guidance (Lunar)

When the lunar svara is active, it's recommended to eat very hot foods, along with sour and pungent dishes and fresh greens, while avoiding cold foods or things that can leave you feeling chilled.

These dietary actions mirror the broader list of actions for the lunar svara. Of course, even if you don't have elephants and aren't practicing archery, many instructions still apply to daily life—when to eat, when to urinate, when to leave the house, and what kind of work to emphasize. I invite you to reflect on the underlying thread that connects all these recommendations.

The Solar Svara (Right Svara / Piṅgalā Nāḍī)

Having reviewed the actions recommended when the left svara is active, we now turn to those recommended to be done or at least initiated when the right svara is active.

Favorable activities include starting on a long journey, traveling towards the north and the east, stepping out with your right leg first, touching the right side of the face with your right hand in the morning, and taking a journey that involve an uneven number of steps. This period is also beneficial for learning or teaching powerful, difficult, or cruel mantras that are used in magic for hurting other people, boarding a ship, interactions between men and women, and engaging in some of the more intense or even the worst and meanest actions described in the text, such as drinking wine or practicing difficult *vīrya* mantras and similar forms of *upāsanā*—intense spiritual *sādhanā*.

The solar svara is linked to states of unrest and agitation and is said to favor acts such as destroying a country, poisoning an enemy, studying the scriptures, traveling, hunting, selling cattle, making bricks, breaking stones, cutting wood, and grinding or polishing gems. It supports physical exercise, overcoming the powers of *yakṣas* and *yakṣiṇīs* (types of demigods), *vetālas* (spirits), ghosts, and poisonous creatures, and riding animals such as donkeys, camels, buffalos, horses, or elephants—remembering that one mounts them with the left svara active, but we ride them with the right svara active. Swimming across rivers or the sea, healing and using medicines, writing letters, killing, attracting or fascinating others, paralyzing or causing hatred amongst people, as well as enchanting and inspiring are also listed here.

Other activities recommended under the solar svara include cultivating land, donating, being enraged and disturbed, buying and selling, calling spirits, performing acts of hostility, and using a sword while fighting the enemy. Enjoying sensual pleasure, having an audience with the king, eating and feasting, bathing—especially taking a cold bath—carrying out general dealings and accomplishing outstanding deeds, gratifying the senses, stimulating the appetite, captivating women, and undertaking all forms of cruel, harsh, and demanding work are also connected with this svara. Additionally, it is considered favorable for tasks requiring dynamism, obtaining knowledge of subtle or difficult-to-access matters, for physical activity more generally, for agriculture and mathematics, and for engaging in opposition, resistance, accusation, or sentencing.

Food Guidance (Solar)

From a dietary perspective, during the solar svara it is recommended to avoid oily foods and refrain from heavy sweet items like sugar, jaggery, milk, and ghee, as well as sour things. An exception is made when sour items are included as part of a balanced meal where sweet things are eaten first, followed by a mixture of sweet and sour, and finally, astringent and bitter things at the end.

The Suṣumṇā / Śūnya Svara (Central Channel)

Finally, we reach the guidance for those times when the breath flows evenly through both nostrils or alternates quickly from one to the other. This pattern indicates that the prāṇa is flowing through the Suṣumṇā nāḍī and is called the Śūnya Svara. Śūnya means emptiness and signifies a state of mind devoid of thoughts and contact with the external world, naturally reducing engagement with the physical world.

This phase is considered highly auspicious for meditation, but it is generally advised to engage only in tasks that require minimal exertion or concentration. The Śūnya Svara is sometimes described as a negative or maleficent svara or nāḍī because any aspirations for material gain or worldly success during this period are said to fail or at least face significant hindrances.

The text even mentions that when someone's time of death is approaching, it's likely to occur during this Svara and it is signaled by having this Svara predominate for extended periods of time. In this sense, the disappearance of the usual nasal cycle can be seen, according to our teaching, as one of the signs of approaching death in someone who is gravely ill or very elderly.

In fact, according to the svara literature, only two types of activities are truly recommended during the Śūnya Svara. The first is *Yoga Abhyāsa* or yogic practices— meditation and any practice through which one wishes to leave the mundane world and act on the spiritual plane. The second encompasses formidable or malevolent actions that require unwavering focus: esoteric, mystical rites and dangerous magical operations that call for an altered state of consciousness and a withdraw from ordinary worldly concerns to be carried out properly.

The *Śiva Svarodaya* offers the following teaching on the Suṣumṇā nāḍī. "If the left Svara flows one moment and the right the next, know thus that Suṣumṇā is flowing. At this time, no action can give worldly profit. Śūnya Svara destroys all action. Then the reason for this is given. The fire element residing in the Suṣumṇā nāḍī burns like the fire of destruction and one should know this fire to be a poison and destroyer of all actions, all worldly actions". Recall that the lunar svara is linked with the moon and its energies, the solar Svara with the energies of the sun, and the Śūnya Svara—the Suṣumṇā—with the fiery energies of Kuṇḍalinī.

The text adds that when both the nāḍīs, Iḍā and Piṅgalā, flow simultaneously in a person, breaking their usual sequences—rather than alternating in a regular rhythm—it is inauspicious. There is no doubt about it. Śiva, who is narrating this text, explains to Pārvatī that "If, in one moment, the breath flows through the left svara and the very next moment through the right, it should be considered irregular and, , the reverse results occur". In other words, if you're trying to achieve something—such as buying a house or attempting to win something—while the Śūnya Svara is active, you may receive the opposite results of what you intend.

"According to the wise, when both the nāḍīs flow together, it is like poison. All actions, good or bad, should be avoided because whatever work is done gives no result". Here the text refers specifically to worldly, mundane work, because this phase is meant for spiritual work.

The *Śiva Svarodaya* explains that: "There is no alternative but to pray to God if the question of life and death, profit or loss, victory or defeat arises, or if one has to face an odd or adverse situation during the flow of

Suṣumṇā", that during this flow there is no way to achieve your goals except by the grace of the Divine. You cannot force nature, so to speak, to give you what you want. This is considered an inauspicious time for worldly effort, and so the only meaningful recourse is spiritual means. "People seeking victory, gain, or pleasure should then concentrate on the Lord of the Universe and should engage exclusively in yogic practices".

The text further advises that during the changeover of Svara —or when the tattvas combine—no auspicious work like acquiring virtues or giving donations should be undertaken. When the uneven svara flows, one is cautioned not even to think of traveling, as it is said to indicate likely trouble on the journey, potential harm, and sometimes even death. In this context, Mukti (liberation) means spiritual practices, while Bhukti (enjoyment) may include the sensual enjoyments of tantric union, which are also treated as forms of spirituality and may be recommended under these conditions.

When prāṇa flows inside of the Suṣumṇā nāḍī, the type of karma activated is the Sāttvik karma— the karma that leads us out of the world rather than deeper into it. And so, it's not considered useful to rely on this svara for worldly accomplishments. For meditators, in fact, Śūnya Svara is the best Svara, the most supportive state: many Haṭha yoga practices are specifically designed so that, just before meditation, your breath enters the Suṣumṇā nāḍī. That's why we have the alternate nostril breathing and many of Kuṇḍalinī mudrās that are designed aim to alternate between the two sides so that the breath "falls" into the center, into the Suṣumṇā, where higher states of consciousness can emerge.

So in fact, Śūnya Svara is the best svara for meditation. So you may ask, why, then, does the text call it the Maleficent or Evil Svara? The answer is that this text, the *Śiva Svarodaya* and the teachings of Svara Yoga in general focus on aligning our actions to the worldly field—not only meditation. Practically speaking, when your breath is equal in both nostrils, or alternates quickly between left and right, it signals that the

Suṣumṇā nāḍī is active, that the Śūnya Svara is active, and this is an ideal time for meditation, while other svaras are better suited to the worldly activities connected with each of them.

In another passage, the *Śiva Svarodaya* reads: "The middle channel, Suṣumṇā, is cruel and wicked in all activities. During the flow of Suṣumṇā, those actions leading to *Bhukti*, meaning sensual enjoyment, and Mukti, liberation, should be undertaken".

This sums the advice the Svara Śastra prescribes for aligning our actions with each of the svaras in order to maximize the potential of our actions, but is this just a spiritual idea or does it have any scientific basis? The answer to this question is the subject of our next chapter.

Chapter 10
The Secret Scientific Basis of Svara Yoga Revealed

Following the guidance of Svara Yoga on which actions should and should not be undertaken during each svara, a conceptualization emerges that aligns with familiar ideas: the Solar Svara on the right side is framed as masculine and yang, while the Lunar Svara on the left is framed as feminine and yin.

When the traditional advice of Svara Yoga is analyzed closely, the Lunar Nāḍī appears consistently associated with qualities which are considered yin—feminine, receptive, soft, submissive, and similar attributes traditionally related to femininity. On the other side, the Solar Svara is considered masculine—harsh, intense, active, outward-moving, and emissive.

Here, I'm putting aside the discussion of whether femininity and masculinity are just social conventions, if they are respective aspects of womanhood and manhood, or if these distinctions even truly fundamentally exist. The aim is to simply present what the tradition says.

But even putting this debate aside we are still left with an important question: does any of this have real merit? Is there a valid scientific explanation or empirical support for this idea that, whether magical or not, breathing through the left nostril correlates with behaviors and events of a more feminine, yin nature? And breathing through the right nostril correlates with more masculine, yang, emissive qualities? This is the question the chapter now turns to explore.

The Two Brain Hemispheres

Of course, the first idea that comes to mind is the fact that the brain has two hemispheres. The right hemisphere is connected to the left side of the body, and the left hemisphere is connected to the right. But does this make the left hemisphere "masculine" because it governs the right side, and the right hemisphere "feminine"? Popular notions claim that the left brain is logical and the right is emotional; that one side is masculine and the other feminine; that one is logical while the other is creative; and even that people can be "left-brained" or "right-brained" in their personality. All of these ideas have been disproven.

There are, however, real and important functional differences between the two hemispheres. When viewed alongside cultural definitions of what it means to be masculine and feminine, some correlation can be seen. Broadly speaking, the right hemisphere tends to look at the bigger picture, while the left hemisphere tends to focus on details. This distinction between thinking sequentially versus thinking in a more parallel or holistic way is probably why people often attribute logical thinking to the left and intuitive thinking to the right. But that oversimplification is not really accurate.

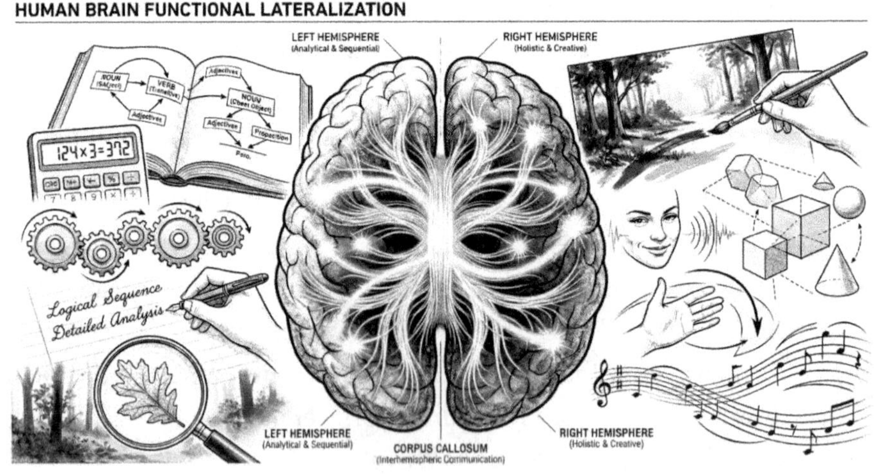

The left side of the brain primarily handles words, while the right side of the brain is more involved with attaching layers of meaning and context to these words. In music, for example, the right side focuses more on melody, whereas the left side focuses on the motor skills needed to produce that melody. In mathematics, the left side performs various calculations like adding, counting, and subtracting, while the right side helps estimate spatial amounts. Spatial orientation in general is definitely a right hemisphere function. Memory tends to be stronger on the left side overall, but negative memories appear particularly tied to right-side processing.

Even in the realm of emotions, negative feelings are more localized to the right hemisphere, which is generally more involved in emotional expression and perception. This side of the brain becomes more active when we try to identify emotional states in ourselves and others. Overactivity in the right hemisphere has been linked to depression, while damage to it can lead to impulsive, quick behavior. There are, without a doubt, meaningful differences between the left and right brain hemispheres.

Connection to the Nervous System

All right, but is there a connection between the nostril through which we are breathing and these left and right brain hemispheres? And what about the parasympathetic and sympathetic branches of the autonomic nervous systems?

If we look at the advice coming from Svara Yoga and compare it to modern knowledge, it definitely appears to echo the lateralization of the brain hemispheres. Even more than that, it corresponds remarkably well to our belief of what is masculine and feminine. However, examining it in depth, the distinction between Solar and Lunar Svara, and what they mean seems to map best onto the division between the parasympathetic "rest and digest" branch and the sympathetic "fight or flight" branch of the autonomic nervous system.

The lunar svara is the calming one, the relaxing one. And the actions recommended to be done on the left svara tend to share those qualities: they are receptive, nourishing, and supportive things that correspond a lot with parasympathetic functioning. By contrast, the actions which are recommended to be performed on the right, solar svara are much more active, proactive, emissive, and outgoing, often requiring a heightened, intense vibration, which aligns closely with the sympathetic nervous system's mobilizing, fight-or-flight role.

The parasympathetic nervous system calms us down and opens the system, making us more receptive, while the sympathetic nervous system agitates and mobilizes us, making us more active and therefore more emissive.

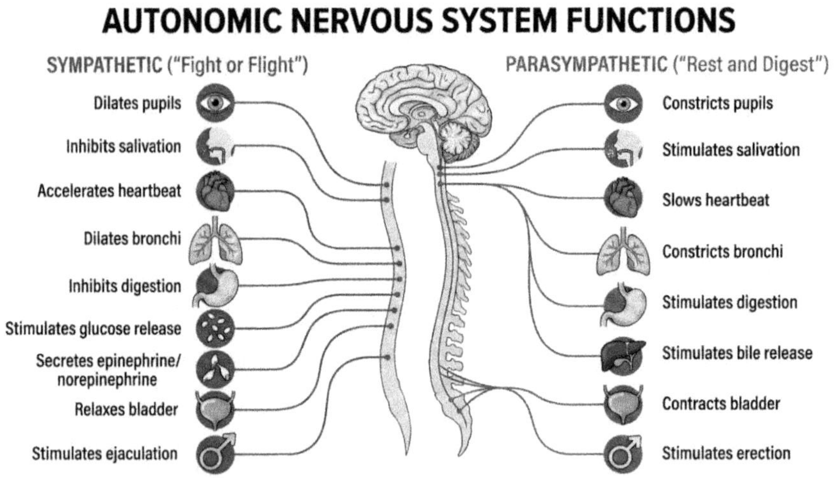

Scientific Correlations

This brings us back to the central question: is there an actual connection between breathing through the left or right nostril, the nasal cycle, the left and right brain hemispheres, and the autonomic nervous system—or is this simply a fanciful yogic idea?

Now, here is the funny thing. At first glance, when superficially reviewing the science, you will likely reach the conclusion that such a direct one-to-one link does not exist. Yet when the research is examined more deeply, you will actually find a more nuanced picture suggesting that connection. It's quite complex from a neurological standpoint. What you will find is that there is a relationship between the nasal cycle dominance, and hemispheric laterality, and that it is this hemispheric laterality, i.e. having one hemisphere more active than the other that determines the relative dominance of either the sympathetic or parasympathetic branches of the nervous system.

Research Findings

A 1983 study showed increased electrical activity in the hemisphere which was contralateral (on the opposite side), to the dominant nostril. Earlier research from1981 indicated that some types of epilepsy could even be triggered by nasal breathing patterns, suggesting that by actively breathing through a single nostril you could might trigger an epileptic event in only one half of the brain.

In 1987, David Shannahoff-Khalsa—a yogi and leading researcher on alternate nostril —demonstrated that by forcibly breathing through either the left or the right nostril, you could cause changes of activation in the contralateral hemisphere.

Continuing his research in 1991, Shannahoff-Khalsa showed that right unilateral forced nostril breathing improved performance on verbal tests, consistent with the understanding that the right nostril activates the left brain hemisphere, which we know is more involved with language. Conversely, forcing the breath to be through the left nostril improved spatial test scores, aligning with the right brain hemisphere's role in spatial processing. Later on, his studies also documented links between nostril dominance and the nature of hallucinations in psychiatric patients, benefits of unilateral forced nostril breathing for speech recovery in stroke patients, and various effects on autonomic balance—or a balance between the sympathetic and parasympathetic nervous systems.

In parallel, research demonstrates that although the control of the autonomic nervous system is mainly distributed and bilateral, there is a slight, but clear and consistent predominance of the left brain hemisphere to increase the activation of the sympathetic branch of the autonomic nervous system, and conversely of the right brain hemisphere to increase the tone in the parasympathetic branch. Put together with the work of David Shannahoff-Khalsa these findings support the conclusion that breathing through the right nostril tends to activate the left brain hemisphere which then increases activity in the sympathetic nervous system, while and breathing through the left nostril tends to activate the right brain which in turn favors the parasympathetic nervous system.

Given this, there definitely is a connection between the nostril through which we are predominantly breathing and the functioning of our brain and nervous system. And I believe that Svara Yoga is largely devoted to exploring and mapping this relationship in detail.

A Scientific Reinterpretation

Svara Yoga traditionally claims that it can predict the future and indicate which actions are likely to succeed based on the active Svara, explaining this in terms of karma and how it flows in each and every moment. But in my vision, without negating this traditional framework, we can offer a parallel and more scientific interpretation focusing on how the active Svara changes our inner state and therefore our behavior in a given situation. In this view, the "success" or "failure" of an action depends less on fate and more on whether our nervous system is in a state that matches what the situation demands. If a situation calls for courage, speed, and sharp focus, having a more sympathetic, right-nostril-dominant state will naturally support more effective action.

Imagine needing to go into battle: Svara Yoga would say you should have the right side active to support successful action and scientifically, I can completely agree with this. If I want to go into battle, into fighting, I want to have my sympathetic nervous system active leading the way and driving me to push forward, rather than be submissive and surrender.

On the other hand, cooking at home, I want to be more parasympathetic, calm and patient because otherwise, I may turn the heat up and burn whatever it is that I'm cooking.

There are nuances, of course. If you are a restaurant chef trying to feed everybody quickly, then a more sympathetic state might be helpful if skillfully channeled. In this case we are talking about the sympathetic nervous system, not necessarily being "sympathetic" to the customers.

Practical Examples

Svara Yoga recommends that when we're making friends, it's better to have the left Svara active, and this is completely logical when viewed through the lens of the nervous system. The parasympathetic system supports social engagement and connection, while the sympathetic system tends to create tension, reactivity, and conflict, which is not what we want when building relationships.

For this reason, in situations like socializing, meeting friends, or visiting a spiritual teacher, it is more helpful to be in a parasympathetic, receptive state rather than a charged, sympathetic one. The sympathetic mode can then be reserved for moments of aggressionI keep for killing, paralyzing others, acts of hostility, right?

Another traditional recommendation is that when we are collecting things, for example, or acquiring land, the left Svara should be active, which is associated with the right brain hemisphere, and greater spatial awareness. And that makes sense. From a modern perspective, this fits well with tasks that require a broader sense of space, context, and environment, where a calmer, more perceptive state can lead to wiser choices.

On Masculinity, Femininity, and Biology

The idea that some qualities are more "masculine" and others "feminine might be rooted in biology, or it might be a social construct. The evidence is mixed and not conclusive. Some ideas suggest that human beings who have two X chromosomes, if left alone, will develop in a way which is what we consider to be feminine.

In the same way, this theory would suggest that if a human being who has one X and one Y chromosome will be left alone, the hormones encoded by that Y chromosome (especially the amount of testosterone) will change how the brain and body is formed in such a way as to produce the qualities we call masculinity.

If this idea if proven to be true (and it has not yet been proven) would serve as the scientific, biological explanation for differences in brain formation and hormonal balance, and therefore behavior between the biological sexes.

However, even when somebody has two X chromosomes, that doesn't necessarily mean that their brain and body will develop in a way that matches what our culture calls feminine, and the same applies to someone has one X chromosome and one Y chromosome. There are factors that can change how the body reacts to the hormones that differentiate between human beings with XX and those with XY chromosomes, in a way that a person with two X chromosomes may develop features and of someone with XY chromosomes, and vice versa, even to the point of not being able to distinguish the two.

And of course XY, and XX are not the only combination of sex hormones, some people have XXX, some have XXY, there's a wide array of how these combinations can manifest. So even within this framework of biology alone there is much more than complexity than a simple dichotomy, but the idea of this theory is that XX chromosomes normally produce what we call feminine traits, and XY chromosomes normally produces what we call masculine.

Other theories relate femininity and masculinity to evolutionary roles, particularly in the theory of the hunter-gatherers. Which suggests that in their role as gatherers and raising children women developed more spatial awareness, more social awareness, and in a sense a more parasympathetic, right-brain affinity, while hunters, which were in the past considered to be mostly men became more sympathetic and more left-brained to be good in the tasks appointed to them. Yet modern research shows that both males and females were involved in both hunting and gathering, even if child rearing was mostly the task of those who could bear children

Moreover, as we have seen the simplistic left-brain/right-brain divide has largely been debunked, and these neat stories do not have solid scientific backing, so we don't even know if any of them are true.

If you're not comfortable with the idea of associating femininity with parasympathetic, right-brained qualities and masculinity with sympathetic, left-brained qualities, you can simply drop that idea. Set it aside. Instead, it is enough to understand that the left, lunar Svara tends to activate the parasympathetic nervous system and the right brain hemisphere, while the right, solar Svara tends to activate the sympathetic nervous system and more of the left brain hemisphere.

Integration of Science and Tradition

Taking all of this into consideration we can conclude that All of the science of Svara Yoga can be distilled into a simple, practical idea: in different events and situations in our lives, it helps to know whether to be more sympathetically activated or more parasympathetically activated. Sometimes we benefit from being a little bit more outgoing, or even a bit aggressive, and at other times it is wiser to be a bit more calm, a bit more inclusive, and a bit more receptive.

When we consciously align the state of our brain and our nervous system with the events around us, our efforts tend to be more effective and less strained. The active Svara then becomes a tool for attuning ourselves: noticing which nostril is dominant and, when needed, gently shifting the flow to support the quality we wish to embody.

For example, if I'm entering a negotiation where strength and assertiveness are crucial, I can activate my sympathetic nervous system by ensuring that the right Svara is flowing as I step into the room. If the right Svara is not active, Svara Yoga offers methods to change the air flow, or nostril dominance, to activate the right Svara. With this, I can enter the negotiation room and stand my ground.

If, on the other hand, I am entering the negotiating room as a mediator rather than one of the sides , a more parasympathetic state is appropriate. In that case, supporting the left Svara can help me stay inclusive, listen deeply to all sides, and avoid being perceived—often unconsciously—as an aggressor.

Micro-Expressions and Behavior

If you're wondering how shifting yourself into a more sympathetic or parasympathetic state, or into a more left-brain or right-brain mode, could possibly affect the environment, a lot of the answer has to do with what we call micro-expressions, micro-movements, and liminal (subtle) behaviors. These are small signals that stay just under the level of conscious awareness yet influence everyone around you, even though nobody can quite place their fingers on it.

If I am the active force in a situation, my inner state will naturally change how I behave in the situation, which direction I move in, and—just as importantly—how others react to me. In Svara Yoga terms, changing the active Svara shifts your nervous system, which then shifts your body language, tone of voice, timing, and presence in ways that quietly recalibrate the whole interaction.

For instance, if I want to ask a favor of someone, it is usually wiser to come from a parasympathetic state, supported by breathing in through the left nostril. If you are interacting with an animal that responds better to a calm person, then I should be parasympathetic. But if it reacts more to clear authority, more sympathetic activation may be appropriate.

And of course, if the Svara keeps shifting— right to left, right to left, without settling—it can create a kind of neutral state that is just not leaning in any certain direction, worse still it can create a feeling of instability and unpredictability of behaviors. For actions that ask a person to be clearly one way or another, this can feel incongruent. The system is neither distinctly sympathetic nor distinctly parasympathetic, and the inner signal is more mixed than focused. That's why traditional Svara Yoga recommends avoiding polarized actions that require a person to be either very receptive or very emissive, very aggressive or very calm. Save these actions for times when the Svara, and your nervous system, are more clearly aligned.

Conclusion

This, then, is the scientific framework that can serve as a basis for understanding Svara Yoga. Does this awareness diminish from the mysticism of Svara Yoga? Perhaps a little, but it does not need to negate the mysticism and the ideas of having nāḍīs and prāṇa and karma flowing through these subtle channels.

My belief and how I teach is that all these levels coexist at the same time. Even if there is some kind of magical karma shaping our destiny, it still must manifest in the physical world, and it does so through our interactions with people, and how they respond to our parasympathetic and sympathetic subliminal behaviors.

Chapter 11

Navigating Nervous System Overdrive: Finding Balance Amid Sympathetic and Parasympathetic Dominance

The Need for Change in the Svara

One of the recurring themes in Svara Yoga is that the Svara is meant to change and not remain fixed in one nostril for too long. The traditional texts describe in multiple places what is believed to happen if the Svara stays constant through a single nostril without changing for extended periods.

For example, the *Śiva Svarodaya,* in verses 331 and 332, says:

> "When the flow of Svara is continuous night and day through one nostril, his death will come in three years.
>
> If the solar Svara of a person flows continuously for two consecutive days and nights, it is said by the knowers of the elements that he has only two years of life remaining.
>
> When the same nāḍī flows continuously for up to three nights, one year is left for him to live, the wise say".

So the yogis noticed that when the flow remains mainly on one side for a long time, something in the physiological system is no longer functioning optimally, and this imbalance can eventually lead to disease and death.

From a modern, scientific standpoint this can be explored as a question about what happens when either the parasympathetic or the sympathetic nervous system is chronically overactivated. Such long-term dominance can create significant difficulties and damages in one's life.

I'm certainly not saying that prolonged overactivation will predict your death in two or three years, but it definitely has some negative effects. To the best of my knowledge, there has been no formal scientific study around what happens if the breath stays only in one nostril for 24 or 48 hours straight. Still, it is reasonable to say that persistent one-sided dominance has negative effects, and the yogic warnings can be read as a poetic yet pointed way of emphasizing the importance of dynamic balance.

Overactivation of the Parasympathetic System

Psychological Effects

What are the psychological and physical difficulties that one may experience when they have a heightened and chronic parasympathetic activation—when one is *too yin*, so to speak?

On the psychological level, one of the first tendencies is excessive passivity. Too much of this so-called calming energy can result in a lack of assertiveness and initiative, potentially creating a sense of powerlessness or being overwhelmed by external circumstances.

This excess can also contribute to a sense of heaviness and sluggishness that can lead to lethargy and apathy, showing as low energy, lack of motivation, and a general disinterest in activities and responsibilities. Over time, this may deepen into chronic depression or a persistent, gray mood.

An overemphasis on introspection and internalizing emotions that arises from this can also lead to emotional imbalance, resulting in excessive sensitivity, moodiness, sadness, and melancholy. Decision-making may become difficult, with a tendency toward indecisiveness and an over-reliance on the guidance of others, instead of trusting one's own direction.

Eventually, this pattern can lead to isolation and withdrawal, a strong preference for solitude and introspection, that may erode social interactions and relationships. Loneliness can then reinforce depressive states, creating a self-perpetuating loop.

Since the right brain hemisphere is more closely connected with negative emotions, excessive dominance on this side can see a rise in anxiety and negative self-interpretations. This often shows up as harsh inner narratives, self-doubt, and a tendency to see oneself and the world through a more pessimistic lens, even though anxiety is also tied to sympathetic activation.

Physical Effects

From a physical standpoint, chronic parasympathetic dominance often shows up first indigestive issues. Heightened parasympathetic activation can lead to increased activity in the digestive system. In excess, this may result in symptoms like frequent bloating, excessive gas, and diarrhea.

It may also cause the metabolic rate to slow, making weight gain more likely and losing weight more difficult. A decrease in heart rate and blood pressure can contribute to dizziness, lightheadedness, and headaches, especially when standing up or exerting yourself.

Cognitive function can be impaired, leading to a sense of mental fog, difficulty concentrating, and a lack of clarity. And finally, difficulty in physical activity itself—low muscle tone, reduced vigor, and lack of motivation for exercise, which together lead to a decline in overall physical fitness.

These patterns are some of what we may experience when the parasympathetic the overly active "rest and digest" branch of our autonomic nervous system is overactive. From a yogic perspective, they are invitations to gently rebalance toward more vitality, engagement, and equilibrium.

Overactivation of the Sympathetic System

Psychological Effects

Having explored parasympathetic excess, let's now look at what happens when we have chronically high sympathetic activation. In this state, the system behaves as if life is a continuous emergency, rather than a rhythm of effort and rest.

On a psychological level, too much sympathetic activation often shows up as restlessness and an agitated mind. This can manifest as an inability to relax, constant fidgeting, and a persistent feeling of inner turmoil.

This heightened drive can fuel impulsive behavior and a lack of patience, leading to hasty decision-making and acting without thorough consideration. Emotional responses tend to become more intense, particularly those of anger, irritability, and anxiety, along with a sense of being constantly in a fight and need to either run away from or confront an imaginary danger, which if left unresolved may develop into generalized anxiety or even panic disorder.

This reactivity easily spills into conflicts with others and a general sense of emotional volatility. In more extreme cases, it can show up as angry outbursts or even increased tendencies toward violence.

Overstimulation and hyperactivity are also common: The mind and body feel amped up, with racing thoughts and a strong need for constant engagement or stimulation. This makes it harder to sit down, concentrate, or sustain attention, and can lead to patterns associated with ADHD (Attention Deficit Hyperactivity Disorder).

Relaxation and sleep are often impacted as well—either a difficulty in falling asleep, staying asleep, or unwinding when there is time to rest. Taken together, all of this can lead to various problems in delaying gratification, strained relationships, and much more.

Physical Effects

On a physical level, chronic hyperactivation of the sympathetic nervous system can show up as increased heart rate and elevated blood pressure. Over time, this raised baseline can lead to cardiovascular strain and a heightened risk of heart-related conditions.

Digestive activity often slows down in this state, since the body is prioritizing "fight or flight" over "rest and digest". This may appear as reduced appetite, constipation, or a persistent feeling of "butterflies" or tightness in the stomach.

Increased muscle tension is another hallmark, with ongoing stiffness and pain, particularly in the neck, shoulders, and back. The presence of excess stress molecules in the bloodstream can lead to various autonomic disorders, allergies, autoimmune issues, chronic inflammation, and conditions such as fibromyalgia and migraine.

There may also be increased sweating and difficulty regulating body temperature, as if the internal thermostat is stuck on high. In some cases, the immune system becomes suppressed, causing one to be more susceptible to frequent illness and infections.

The Importance of Balance

It's clear that being tilted toward parasympathetic or sympathetic overactivity is not supportive of a healthy, integrated life. What Svara

Yoga emphasizes again and again is the need for balance between the active and calming branches of the nervous system.

In the next chapter, we'll explore practical techniques for shifting the active Svara from one nostril to the other. These methods allow you to influence your state, align the Svara with your intended actions to get maximum rewards for your efforts, and how to rebalance when one side has been chronically active for too long.

Chapter 12
Mastering Nasal Cycle Shifting Techniques: How to Change the Dominant Nostril at Will

Imagine yourself before an important business negotiation where you know you must be clear and strong. You must be assertive. You need to be in charge. The meeting starts at 11 A.M. in five minutes. As you check your breath, you realize that it is predominantly flowing on the left side.

You remember the teachings of Svara Yoga, and recognize entering a negotiation of this sort with the lunar Svara active is not ideal if you want to be assertive and get specific outcomes. For a situation that calls for confident, forward-moving energy, a more sympathetic state and an active solar Svara would serve you much better. In the moment, you contemplate your actions. What can you do? Should you postpone the meeting and wait for your body to naturally shift to the right Svara?

The reassuring answer is No. You are not abandoned to the mercy of the spontaneous nasal cycle. Svara Yoga teaches us practical methods to physically manipulate and shift the active Svara from one nostril to another. These techniques usually take about five to fifteen minutes to take effect, giving you a realistic window to adjust your inner state before stepping into action.

So let's see what you can do to actually shift your Svara. In the following sections, you will explore how to apply these methods so that you can consciously align your Svara with your intentions and the demands of the moment. In this way, the breath becomes not only a mirror of your state, but also a tool for skillful, embodied choice.

Technique 1 – Closing the Active Nostril and breathing in through the Inactive nostril

The first and simplest method for shifting the Svara is to mechanically close the nostril that is active. This gently forces the body to breathe through the opposite nostril and begins the shift toward the opposite Svara.

So, for example, if you're breathing predominantly through the left nostril and you want to activate the solar Svara, you can simply close the left nostril with your finger, a small piece of cotton, or even an ear plug—which actually works surprisingly well, funny as it may sound. By simply blocking the active nostril and breathing normally, you force the flow to move to the other side.

Now, of course, the nervous system does not flip instantly. Closing the right nostril will not immediately activate the lunar Svara. It usually takes about five to ten minutes, for the deeper shift to occur, even though the physical airflow changes right away.

This is a highly effective option if you need to immediately shift to another Svara. This is one of the key techniques I employ with clients to alleviate migraine attacks that are triggered by a chronic sympathetic activation followed by depletion of neurotransmitters used by this system. Closing the right nostril and breathing only through the left when the signs of an impending attack appear can, in some cases, completely prevent the attack.

This has been especially helpful for athletes such as are soccer and football players who tend to get migraine attacks after the intense physical exertion involved in their sport. Some of them simply plug the right nostril in the locker room after the game as they are getting ready, and after thirty minutes or so of breathing through the left side, they usually manage to avert the migraine attack altogether.

This is a great method because once the nostril is plugged, you don't need to do anything else. The device stops the breathing, sets the pattern, and the body follows. The only drawback is that it might not be appropriate for every situation—most people don't want to walk into a business meeting with a pink or yellow earplug sticking out of one nostril.

But even if you cannot keep your nostril plugged all the time breathing through the inactive or partly clogged nostril—the inactive Svara—encourages it to become more dominant, and can help shift the svara within a few minutes.

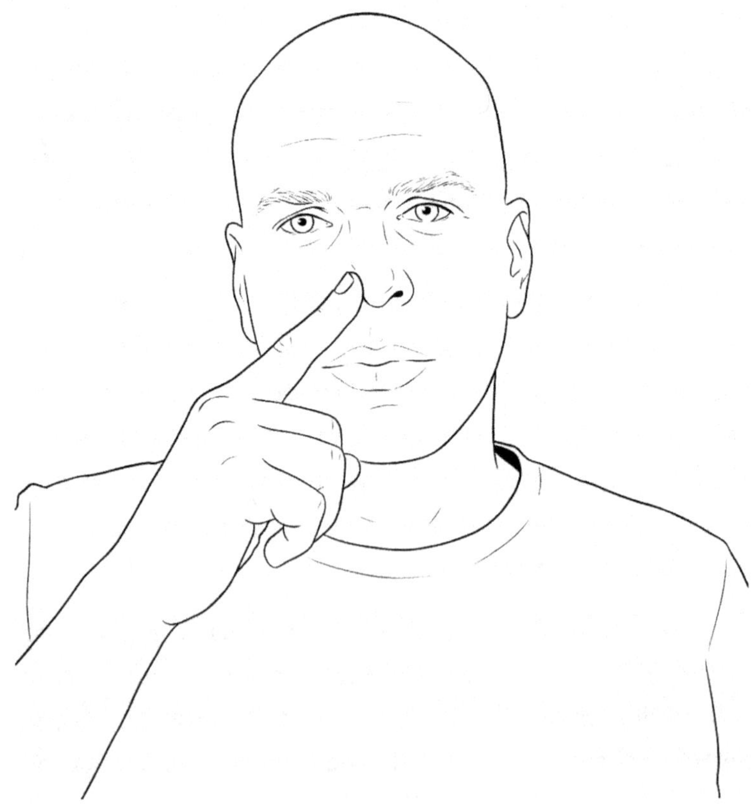

Technique 2 – Inhale Through the Inactive Nostril and Exhale through the Active Nostril

Traditional Svara Yoga teaches that in order to induce a shift from one svara to another one should inhale through the clogged nostril (the inactive Svara) and exhale through the active Svara.

So, if you're currently breathing freely through the right nostril and you want to shift to the left, you inhale through the left and exhale through the right until the balance changes.

Conversely, if your left nostril is free and active and you want more breath to pass through the right, inhale through the right nostril and exhale through the left. Practiced for several minutes, this pattern gently invites the inactive side to wake up and take the lead.

Medical research suggests that the key biological mechanism involved in the nasal cycle sits in the upper part of the nasal cavity and is primarily triggered by inhalation. So, as long as you inhale through the inactive Svara—the congested side with less airflow—it doesn't really matter whether you exhale through the same nostril, the opposite nostril, or even through the mouth.

But if you want to stay close to the classical method, the Svara Yoga way, you would inhale through the inactive Svara, the slightly congested nostril, and exhale through the nostril with more air.

Technique 3 – Pressure Points Under the Armpits

Technique number three uses a unique pressure point under the armpit that, when pressed, activates the opposite Svara.

The key principle to remember is simple: press on the side of the active Svara that is opposite to the side you want to open.

So, if you're currently breathing in mainly through the left nostril and want to be breathing through the right, make a fist with your right hand. Lift your left elbow out to the side, like lifting a chicken wing, and place your fist into the armpit, pressing a slightly upward as if you're trying to push the elbow higher.

Then slowly bring the left elbow down so it wraps around and engulfs your right fist deep inside of the armpit, drawing the left elbow to the side of the body. You can use your left hand to grab hold of your right elbow and gently pull, increasing the pressure of the fist into the left armpit.

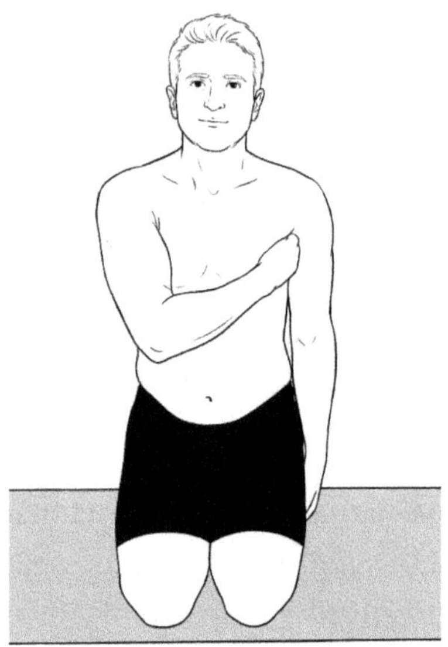

Just staying like this, with steady pressure for five to ten minutes, usually shifts the breath from being left-side dominant to right-side dominant.

In other words, by pressing on the side that is active, you shift activation to the other side. Here, you're using your right fist in the left armpit to shift the Svara from an active lunar Svara to an active solar Svara—from having a free left nostril to a freer right nostril.

And if the right nostril is active and you want open the left, simply reverse the sides: make a fist with the left hand, place it under the right armpit, press up, bring the right elbow down, and use the right palm to pull the left elbow so the fist presses more deeply. This reliably shifts the breath from the right to the left.

This is considered a highly effective and practical method.

A Note from the *Kālacakra Tantra*:

The *Kālacakra Tantra*, even suggests that we add an element: pinch the nipple on the same, active side while pressing into the armpit—the left nipple with left armpit pressure, or right nipple with right armpit pressure—to enhance the effect.

Technique 4 – Lying on the Active Side

If applying pressure feels like too much effort or isn't appropriate for the situation, our fourth technique for shifting the breath from one nostril to another is simply to lie down on the same side as the active Svara.

If the open nostril is on the right, and you want to switch it to the left lie down on your right side, with the left side facing up, using gravity and the weight of the body rather than direct manipulation to compress the active side and leaving the left side free to open. In this way the breath will slowly shift to be active on the left side. Over several minutes, the left nostril usually begins to open and the dominant flow gradually shifts, moving from the solar Svara to the lunar Svara.

You can also combine this position with any of the previous three techniques. For example, while lying on your right side to shift toward the left nostril, apply armpit pressure, or use the breathing pattern—inhaling through the left and exhaling through the right—or you even use a nose plug.

The same logic applies in reverse: if your left nostril is currently active and you want awaken the right, lie on your left side so the right side is facing up. From there, you can add whichever of the earlier methods is most comfortable and context-appropriate to support the shift.

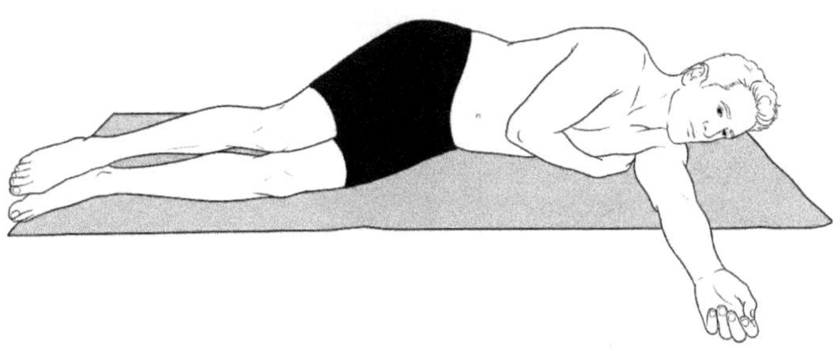

Technique 5 – Sudden Temperature Change

Finally, there are a few more tricks that don't necessarily target a specific nostril, but simply cause a shift in the Svara. One of the most accessible methods is exposing yourself to a sudden, strong temperature contrast— That can be done by applying either very cold or very hot water or air, anything that is remarkably different from your physical experience in that moment. The shift in temperature tends to diminish the difference between the nostrils even to the point of bringing them into an apparent momentary equilibrium, from which you can use the other techniques to shift the nasal cycle in the direction you prefer.

If you did want to apply this technique to induce a specific change modern research has shown that the left nostril is more sensitive and becomes more active in response to warming sensations, and the right nostril to cooling sensations. So if you wanted to shift from a lunar to a solar svara, from left to right you can induce it through applying very cold water to your face, and if you wanted to do the reverse, by applying warm water.

Technique 6 – Using Diet to Influence the Svara

Diet is also thought to affect the overall parasympathetic and sympathetic balance. And while I do agree that these diet-based strategies work, because digestion unfolds over many hours, I don't find diet a very efficient for working with Svara Yoga in the moment. It is better viewed as a long-term way to balance our sympathetic and parasympathetic nervous systems generally, rather than a sharp instrument for quickly shifting the active nostril.

Foods that Activate the Sympathetic (Heating) Response

Certain "warming" foods tend to stimulate the body and are associated with increased sympathetic activation. These include:

Fruits: apricots, bananas, cantaloupe, cherries, cranberries, grapes, grapefruit, kiwi, lemon, oranges, papaya, peaches, pineapple, plums, tamarind.

Vegetables: artichoke, Brussels sprouts, carrots, chilies, corn, dandelion, eggplant, leeks, mushrooms, mustard greens, olives, onions, bell peppers, radishes, spinach, squash, tomatoes, turnips.

Grains: buckwheat, corn, millet, rice, rye, spelt.

Legumes and Nuts: kidney beans, brown lentils, miso, tempeh, almonds, Brazil nuts, cashew nuts, macadamia nuts, peanuts, pecans, pistachios, walnuts.

Meats: beef, chicken, duck, lamb, pork.

Spices and Drinks: chili, cinnamon, garlic, ginger, mustard, pepper, alcohol, black tea, coffee.

All of these will increase the activation of the sympathetic nervous system.

Foods that Activate the Parasympathetic (Cooling) Response

On the other hand, cooling foods are linked with a calming, parasympathetic response. These include:

Fruits: apples, melons, pears, prunes, strawberries, watermelon.

Vegetables: sprouts, cucumber, celery, cauliflower, cabbage, broccoli, beets, okra, peas.

Grains and Legumes: barley, oats, tapioca, black-eyed peas, adzuki beans, mung beans, almonds, coconut.

Milk Products: milk, buttermilk, yogurt.

Drinks: chamomile tea, coconut water, lemon water, peppermint tea.

While all these foods are said to have a cooling influence, you can search online and find multiple lists. Some will contradict each other, but experiment, observe your own reactions, and find a personal balance that works for your system.

Exploring Further

These dietary ideas can accompany the Svara-shifting methods you have learned, offering another way to influence sympathetic–parasympathetic balance over time. I invite you to try out these exercises, note your experiences, and even discover new variations that suit your unique body-mind.

Beyond controlling the Svara, future chapters will look at aligning daily activities around your breath from the moment you wake up, balancing the sympathetic and parasympathetic nervous systems more broadly, and moving into deeper synchronization with astrological cycles.

Chapter 13
Harmonizing Daily Life by Embracing the Svara Rhythms

Now that the foundations of Svara are in place, the next step is to weave this awareness into the flow of an ordinary day. The practice begins from the very first moments after waking, turning simple actions into conscious, breath-aligned choices.

Beginning the Day with Awareness

Upon waking, we first want to identify which Svara is active. Once you recognize it, lightly touch that side of the head with the corresponding hand—for example, if the lunar Svara is active rest the left palm on the left side of your head.

Next, as you step out of bed, let the foot that matches the active Svara touch the ground first. If your solar Svara is active and the right nostril is dominant, step forward with your right foot, ideally moving towards the east or north. If the lunar Svara is active and the left channel is more open, step first with your left foot first, turning toward the west or south.

Morning Activities Aligned with the Svara

If you plan to take a cold shower, it is best to do so when the solar Svara is active, and if you want to take a warm shower, do it when the lunar Svara is flowing.

When you approach breakfast, check your Svara again and let it guide your food choices. If the solar Svara is active, avoid hot, pungent, sour, and oily foods and learn toward cooling options. If the lunar Svara is active, skip the cooling foods and opt for warming ones instead.

When you are about to go to the toilet, notice which Svara is active. If the left Svara is dominant, this is a good sign of health and balance, whereas an active right Svara at this time can mean that stress is running high.

Interactions and Movement Throughout the Day

When leaving for work, school, or wherever you need to go, make sure to step out of the house with the foot that corresponds to the active Svara. As you walk through the day and meet people—especially if you hope to approach someone in a friendly way after some prior conflict—take the first step toward them with the same-side foot as the active nostril and keep your inactive side facing them during the interaction.

If you need to issue instructions or assert authority, position yourself so the other person stands on the side of your active Svara.

Traditional teachings also note that when femininity wants to attract masculinity, it is important to keep the other on the side of a flowing lunar Svara, and when masculinity wants to attract femininity, to keep the feminine on the side of an active solar Svara.

Whenever you give or receive anything, use the hand that corresponds to the currently active Svara, letting even simple exchanges become part of your breath-based alignment.

Balancing Activity and Receptivity

Check your Svara throughout the day, and keep returning to the simple question: what does this moment ask of me—activity or receptivity. When you need to be dynamic, leading, or outwardly engaged, it is helpful to shift the Svara to be more active on the solar, right side. When you need to soften or take a supporting role, shift your Svara to the lunar, left side.

These moment-to-moment adjustments sit on top of a larger principle from the Svarodaya Śāstra: maintaining harmony between the warm, solar breath of the right nāḍī and the cool, lunar breath of the left nāḍī. In this way, both the physical and subtle bodies are cared for, and neither pole dominates for too long.

Balancing Practices for Day and Night

Traditional teachings also offer guidelines that link Svara practice with the lunar cycle. During the illumined phase of the lunar month, when the moon is waxing and governs the night, it's considered beneficial to block the left nostril while sleeping so that only the right channel flows, helping to restore equilibrium.

In the dark half of the month, when the moon's influence diminishes, the recommendation is reversed: block the right, sun channel at night and let the lunar nāḍī flow freely throughout the night.

If at any point—particularly while walking or engaging in physical activities—you experience a sudden rise in body temperature or a wave of extreme fatigue, it's considered beneficial to block the right nostril and allow the breath to flow only through the left nostril until the system settles again.

Preserving Prāṇa and Energetic Balance

Traditional Svarodaya texts describe how, during very cold or very hot days, various types of prāṇa can escape through the minor channels *Puṣā* and *Yasasvinī* that pass through the ears. To preserve prāṇa, it is recommended to cover the ears in both extremes of temperatures, protecting the subtle as well as the physical body.

Another support for energetic balance is meditation: visualizing a bright full moon resting between the eyebrows is believed to soothe psychosomatic disturbances and maintain a cool, clear, refreshed state of mind.

Traditional Health-Related Advice

When intense thirst arrives without available water, some teachings suggest closing the right nostril and meditating on the tongue, sensing saliva gently dripping onto it. This practice is considered to ease the feeling of thirst until water can be found.

Finally, after eating, some *Svarodaya* texts recommend practicing just two minutes of alternate nostril prāṇāyāma. This brief balancing of the channels is believed to support digestion, helping both body and breath to process the meal with greater ease.

Chapter 14
The Svara and the Stars: How Astrology and the Science of Svara Combine

The study of Svara Yoga is intimately connected with the study of Vedic or Indian Astrology (*Jyotiṣa*). The *Śiva Svarodaya* even claims that astrology without the science of Svara is essentially useless..

Beyond the individual flow of Svara in a person, these teachings speak of a cosmic Svara, a universal breath that moves through the planet itself according to the rising and setting of celestial bodies. These planetary movements shift the balance of the five elements and influence the relative dominance of Idā and Piṅgalā, so that personal and cosmic rhythms constantly interweave.

The *Śiva Svarodaya* teaches us how to align our individual Svara, identified through the nostrils, into alignment with this larger universal breath of the cosmos.

Planetary Horas

One of the more subtle ways the ancients perceived time was through what came to be known as *planetary horas*, or planetary hours.

These are not fixed sixty-minute units, but rather variable segments of the day and night, each governed by one of the seven classical planets: Saturn, Jupiter, Mars, the Sun, Venus, Mercury, and the Moon.

Planetary horas are used more explicitly in Western occultism and do not appear directly in the Svara Yoga literature. Still, because they underpin the planetary days employed both in Svara Yoga and in Vedic astrology, I include them here as a useful bridge of understanding, even though you will not see them mentioned in quotations from the *Śiva Svarodaya* itself.

The Nature of Planetary Hours

The ancients divided the sunlit part of the day into twelve equal parts, and the night into another twelve. Since the lengths of day and night shift throughout the year, these planetary hours naturally expand and contract with the seasons. Only around the equinoxes, when the length of day and night are equal, does a planetary hour last exactly sixty minutes.

At other times they vary in length: In winter, daytime planetary hours are shorter than 60 minutes and nighttime hours are longer, while in summer this pattern reverses: longer planetary hours by day and shorter ones by night.

Calculating Your Planetary Hours

To calculate planetary hours for a specific location and date:

1. Find local sunrise and sunset times for the specific date.
2. Calculate the day length by subtracting sunrise from sunset.
3. Divide that span by 12 to get the length of one daytime planetary hour.
4. Subtract the day length from 24 hours to find the night length.
5. Divide that by 12 to get the length of one nighttime planetary hour.

Example: In Amsterdam on December 27:

- Day length: 7 hours 42 minutes (7.7 hours)
- Daytime planetary hour: 7.7 ÷ 12 = 38 minutes

- Night length: 16 hours 18 minutes (16.3 hours)
- Nighttime planetary hour: 16.3 ÷ 12 = 82 minutes

Near the equator, as in India, where day and nights remain close to 12 hours year-round, planetary hours remain close to 60 minutes almost all the time.

The Chaldean Order

Each planetary hour is ruled by one of the seven classical planets, following an order known as the Chaldean Order. This order, inherited by the Babylonians from the Chaldeans, went on to influence most Eastern and Western systems of astrology.

The Chaldean order is based on the apparent speed of the seven visible heavenly bodies as seen from Earth, from slowest to fastest:

Saturn → Jupiter → Mars → Sun → Venus → Mercury → Moon.

This sequence also reflects how the ancient Babylonians imagined their distances , with Saturn farthest away and the Moon nearest, so that moving through the order from Saturn back to the Moon traces a descent from outermost to innermost. Once the Moon is reached, the cycle returns again to Saturn and repeats.

The Seven Planets and Their Influences

Each planet is understood to carry its own energetic signature that colors both circumstances and internal states. By understanding these qualities, one can choose activities that resonate more naturally with a given planetary hour.

Saturn (Śani) — The Disciplinarian

Saturn represents discipline, responsibility, and structure, bringing the energy of endurance, practicality, and long-term planning. It is linked with setting limits, exercising self-control, completing cycles, and, in Western astrology, with the slow winding down that precedes renewal.

In the Indian tradition, Saturn also represents sustained hard work that leads to lasting success, while at the same time being associated with obstacles and the ripening of difficult karma. Therefore, Śani hour is best approached with care and is especially suitable for tapas (austerities), meditation, fulfilling duties, and finishing or releasing what needs to be brought to a close.

Jupiter (Guru) — The Expander

Jupiter governs expansion, optimism, wisdom, abundance, and growth, bringing a sense of insight, generosity, and abundance to whatever it touches. In some traditions it is also considered as the planet of savings and accumulation, supporting steady increase over time.

In the Indian tradition, Jupiter is the guru, the teacher and spiritual guide, enhancing wisdom, knowledge, optimism, generosity, and spirituality. Jupiter presides over education, wealth, growth, and spiritual development, and brings prosperity to whatever he touches. Jupiter's hours are especially supportive for studying, teaching, learning, long-term planning, investments, and rituals or blessings.

Mars (Maṅgala) — The Warrior

Mars is connected with action, courage, assertiveness, ambition, and physical vitality, and governs protection, defense, and strategic response. Mars is strongly associated with resolving conflicts—sometimes diplomatically, sometimes through more direct and forceful means.

In the Indian tradition, Mars is highly competitive and, when skillfully channeled, can drive success in career and personal endeavors. Mars hours are excellent for exercise, taking initiative, setting and defending boundaries, confronting challenges, and acting decisively, though there is a need to watch for unnecessary aggression or impulsive haste.

The Sun (Sūrya) — The Illuminator

The Sun radiates vitality, confidence, self-expression, and creativity and is associated with leadership, individuality, health, beauty, poetry, music, and divination. When solar energy is excessive, it can lead to ego-driven behavior, overshadowing subtler or more relational qualities.

In Indian astrology, the Sun governs the self and ego, the father, and one's public role or career, and its activation often brings visibility and recognition. Sun hours are ideal for launching important projects, meeting authority figures, seeking recognition, strengthening health practices, and stepping into leadership or creative expression.

Venus (Śukra) — The Harmonizer

Beautiful Venus is associated with love, beauty, sensuality, harmony, relationships, and artistic expression. She governs aesthetic appreciation, emotional connection, companionship, sensual pleasures, and the enjoyment of material comfort.

In the Indian tradition, Venus also rules luxury, creativity, and refined, harmonious relationships. Venus hours are especially supportive for meeting loved ones, creating art, enjoying beauty, reconciling differences, preparing or enjoying food, romance, and simple sensual rest —while remembering Venus's shadow of indulgence, laziness, and escapism.

Mercury (Budha) — The Messenger

Mercury governs communication, commerce, transactions, travel, technology, language, writing, learning, wit, and mental agility. As the messenger of the gods, Mercury influences clarity of thought, intelligence, eloquence, and, in some traditions, even magic itself.

Mercury hours are excellent for reading, studying, writing, negotiating, planning, managing correspondence, and teaching. If explaination something feels difficult or technology is oddly uncooperative, check whether Mercury's hour is approaching—the shift can be remarkable.

The Moon (Candra) — The Nurturer

The Moon is connected to the lunar energies of emotion, intuition, receptivity, nurturing, instincts, and the subconscious or unconscious mind. She embodies the ever-changing face of the divine feminine and invites the exploration of subtle, hidden aspects of oneself, including the mystical and the magical.

In Indian astrology, the Moon is linked with home, domestic life, and mothers, and has a strong influence on mental stability and emotional well-being. Moon hours are ideal for family matters, social connection, rest, self-care, emotional healing, and intuitive practices, offering a space to tend loved ones and listen more deeply to the subtle currents of feeling.

Planetary Hours Quick Reference Table

Planet	Nature	Best for	Avoid / Caution	Svara Alignment
Sun	Vital, authoritative, clarifying	Begin important projects, seek recognition, meet authority figures, strengthen health, leadership or creative expression	Ego-driven conflict, pride, overexertion	Piṅgalā (Right nostril) — solar, outward, active
Moon	Energetic, assertive, protective	Exercise, take initiative, defend boundaries, confront challenges, act decisively	Aggression, haste, injury	Piṅgalā (Right nostril) — fiery, decisive, dynamic

Planet	Nature	Best for	Avoid / Caution	Svara Alignment
Mercury	Quick, intellectual, communicative	Study, write, teach, negotiate, plan, handle correspondence, travel	Overthinking, gossip, nervous tension	Balanced / Either — harmonizes solar and lunar
Venus	Harmonizing, affectionate, aesthetic	Meet loved ones, create art, enjoy beauty, reconcile, cook, romance, sensual experiences	Indulgence, laziness, escapism	Idā (Left nostril) — soft, relational, cooling
Mars	Energetic, assertive, protective	Exercise, take initiative, defend boundaries, confront challenges, act decisively	Aggression, haste, injury	Piṅgalō (Right nostril) — fiery, decisive, dynamic
Jupiter	Expansive, generous, wise	Teach, learn, travel, invest, plan long-term goals, blessings, rituals, prosperity	Over-confidence, wastefulness, excess	Balanced / Slightly Solar — outward growth with clarity
Saturn	Disciplined, organizing, purifying	Structure work, clean, budget, fulfill duties, complete or release what's finished, meditation, fasting	Pessimism, rigidity, withdrawal	Idā → Piṅgalā transition — grounding, stabilizing, inward discipline leading to outward clarity

Complete Planetary Hours Table

In the table below you can find the complete order of the planetary hours for the entire week.

Hour	Sunday (Sun)	Monday (Moon)	Tuesday (Mars)	Wednesday (Mercury)	Thursday (Jupiter)	Friday (Venus)	Saturday (Saturn)
1 (Sunrise)	Sun	Moon	Mars	Mercury	Jupiter	Venus	Saturn
2	Venus	Saturn	Sun	Moon	Mars	Mercury	Jupiter
3	Mercury	Jupiter	Venus	Saturn	Sun	Moon	Mars
4	Moon	Mars	Mercury	Jupiter	Venus	Saturn	Sun
5	Saturn	Sun	Moon	Mars	Mercury	Jupiter	Venus
6	Jupiter	Venus	Saturn	Sun	Moon	Mars	Mercury
7	Mars	Mercury	Jupiter	Venus	Saturn	Sun	Moon
8	Sun	Moon	Mars	Mercury	Jupiter	Venus	Saturn
9	Venus	Saturn	Sun	Moon	Mars	Mercury	Jupiter
10	Mercury	Jupiter	Venus	Saturn	Sun	Moon	Mars
11	Moon	Mars	Mercury	Jupiter	Venus	Saturn	Sun
12	Saturn	Sun	Moon	Mars	Mercury	Jupiter	Venus
(Sunset) 1	Jupiter	Venus	Saturn	Sun	Moon	Mars	Mercury
2	Mars	Mercury	Jupiter	Venus	Saturn	Sun	Moon
3	Sun	Moon	Mars	Mercury	Jupiter	Venus	Saturn
4	Venus	Saturn	Sun	Moon	Mars	Mercury	Jupiter
5	Mercury	Jupiter	Venus	Saturn	Sun	Moon	Mars
6	Moon	Mars	Mercury	Jupiter	Venus	Saturn	Sun
7	Saturn	Sun	Moon	Mars	Mercury	Jupiter	Venus
8	Jupiter	Venus	Saturn	Sun	Moon	Mars	Mercury
9	Mars	Mercury	Jupiter	Venus	Saturn	Sun	Moon
10	Sun	Moon	Mars	Mercury	Jupiter	Venus	Saturn
11	Venus	Saturn	Sun	Moon	Mars	Mercury	Jupiter
12 (Next Sunrise)	Mercury (Monday)	Jupiter → (Tuesday)	Venus → (Wednesday)	Saturn → (Thursday)	Sun → (Friday)	Moon → (Saturday)	Mars → (Sunday)

How to Read the Table:

- Hour 1 (Sunrise) = First hour of the day; this planet rules the whole day
- Hour 12 (Sunset) = Transition from day to night
- Hour 1 after sunset begins the night cycle, continuing the same Chaldean sequence
- After 24 hours, the next sunrise begins a new day with the next planet in sequence

Example: Saturday ends with Mars; the next planet is the Sun — hence Sunday begins

Practical Applications: Working with Planetary Hours

The essence of working with planetary hours is learning to move in harmony with the prevailing current of the cosmos. Each hour carries the subtle vibration of one of the seven classical planets, and when actions match that tone, effort feels more like catching the wind in our sails rather than rowing against a heavy tide.

In daily life, this can look very simple:

Communication Challenges: If someone cannot understand what you're trying to explain, note the time and check which planetary hour is active. If it's not Mercury's hour, consider revisiting the conversation then and notice how much more easily it may flow. The difference can be striking.

Technology Troubles: When devices misbehave, checking whether Mercury's hour is near can be surprisingly helpful—sometimes simply waiting for Mercury's influence to arrive can make troubleshooting smoother.

Sending Important Messages: For love notes or sensitive outreach where you hope for a positive response, Venus's hour offers a particularly supportive, relational field.

Social Gatherings: Choose Venus hours for enjoyment, pleasure, and social ease, and Mars hours for strategic, energetic business discussions.

Creative vs. Administrative Work: Moon or Venus hours favor creative, intuitive, or emotional work, while Sun or Mars hours support decisive, leadership-oriented, and administrative tasks.

Physical Exercise: Mars hours are ideal for vigorous training, competition, and pushing physical limits.

Study and Learning: Mercury hours enhance quick learning and information processing; Jupiter hours help with deeper wisdom, philosophy, and long-range understanding.

Life, of course, does not always wait for the perfect planetary hour. Yet when important decisions, conversations, or crucial actions are at stake, aligning them with the appropriate planetary influence can noticeably reduce friction and increase a sense of natural support.

Aligning with Your Svara

In the language of Svara Yoga, these planetary forces correspond to the rhythmic alternation of Piṅgalā and Idā—the solar and lunar flows of prāṇa through the nostrils. The solar Piṅgalā breath supports action, clarity, and assertion, while the lunar Idā breath nurtures receptivity, intuition, and sensitivity.

By tracking the dominant nostril and the ruling planetary hour, a more refined alignment of inner and outer rhythms becomes available. This is where astrology and Svara truly meet—the breath in the body and the "breath" of the cosmos moving together, turning everyday choices into a subtle practice of yoga with time.

During solar, or Piṅgalā, hours—particularly those ruled by the Sun, Mars, or Jupiter— the atmosphere supports decisive movement, ambition, leadership, and the outward projection of will. These are excellent times to begin important tasks, take initiative, enter competition, or make firm decisions that require clarity and drive.

Lunar, or Idā, hours—those under the influence of the Moon, Venus, or Saturn— tend to favor gentleness, reflection, emotional connection, and inward-turning activity. This is a natural window for rest, artistic expression, meditation, domestic matters, or quiet healing; Venus softens, the Moon nourishes, and Saturn stabilizes, all inclining the breath inward and deepening awareness.

Mercury and Jupiter function as bridges between the two poles. Mercury's hours are ideal for communication, study, writing, and planning—times that call for both reflection and clear expression. Jupiter's hours widen the field of understanding and faith, supporting teaching, generosity, and long-term vision. Working consciously with these harmonizing currents allows the Svara practitioner not only to act at the right time, but also to feel that time itself becomes a partner on the path.

Planetary Days

The ancients believed that the first planetary hour after sunrise sets the tone for the entire day. The planet that rules this first hour therefore becomes the ruler of that day itself.

If the Chaldean sequence of planetary hours—Saturn, Jupiter, Mars, Sun, Venus, Mercury, Moon—runs continuously through all twenty-four hour divisions, you will find that the planet governing the first hour on the next day will be three steps forward in the sequence. This progression gives the familiar order of planetary days: Sun (Sunday), Moon (Monday), Mars (Tuesday), Mercury (Wednesday), Jupiter (Thursday), Venus (Friday), and Saturn (Saturday).

In fact, the very names of the days still preserve these associations:

Sunday is literally the day of the Sun, Monday of the Moon; Tuesday comes from Tiw's Day (Tiw being the Germanic counterpart of Mars, just as French Mardi still means "the day of Mars". Wednesday is Mercredi in French (from Mercury), Thursday corresponds to Jeudi (from Jupiter) and to Thor's Day in English is Thursday with Thor echoing Jupiter's role, and Friday is Vendredi in French (from Venus), and Freya's Day in English, named for the goddess of love.

Day	Planet	Nature	Auspicious Dominant Naḍi at sunrise	Qualities
Sunday	Sun (Surya)	Solar	Piṅgalā	Vitality, illumination, expression
Monday	Moon (Candra)	Lunar	Idā	Emotion, receptivity, intuition
Tuesday	Mars (Maṅgala)	Solar	Piṅgalā	Courage, energy, protection
Wednesday	Mercury (Budha)	Lunar	Idā	Communication, intellect, trade
Thursday	Jupiter (Guru)	Lunar	Idā	Expansion, wisdom, generosity
Friday	Venus (Śukra)	Lunar	Idā	Love, harmony, beauty
Saturday	Saturn (Śani)	Solar	Piṅgalā	Discipline, structure, completion

Because, as we saw, some of the planets are considered more lunar and others more solar, certain days lean naturally toward inward, receptive, lunar activities, while others are generally more auspicious for assertive, solar activities. The following table summarizes these correspondences and can be used together with Svara awareness to choose both the right day and the right inner state for different kinds of actions.

So on Sundays, Tuesdays, and Saturdays, actions that correspond to the solar svara—clear, assertive, outward-moving endeavors—tend to be more supported. On Mondays, Wednesdays, Thursdays, and Fridays, activities aligned with the lunar Svara—receptive, relational, reflective movements—generally find more ease and success.

The Lunar Fortnights (Pakṣas)

Moving beyond the weekly rhythm of planetary days, Svara Yoga also teaches us to align with the waxing and waning of the moon. A lunar cycle, termed a lunar month lasts approximately 29.5 solar days and in India is traditionally divided into 30 lunar days, or tithis:

- **15 days of waxing** (Śukla Pakṣa): Starting from the new moon, the Śukla Pakṣa progresses as the Moon slowly grows brighter and fuller in the sky each night until it reaches the full moon.
- **15 days of waning** (Kṛṣṇa Pakṣa): Starting on the full moon, the Kṛṣṇa Pakṣa begins and the Moon gradually diminishes and thins out night by night until it disappears again at the following new moon.

A tithi is defined as the time it takes the Moon to move 12° further from the Sun as seen from Earth. Because both the Moon and Earth are moving, this interval is not constant. It ranges from roughly 19 to 26 hours, making the actual calculation of tithis extremely complicated. Luckily for us, modern tables and apps make it easy to know the exact tithi at any moment.

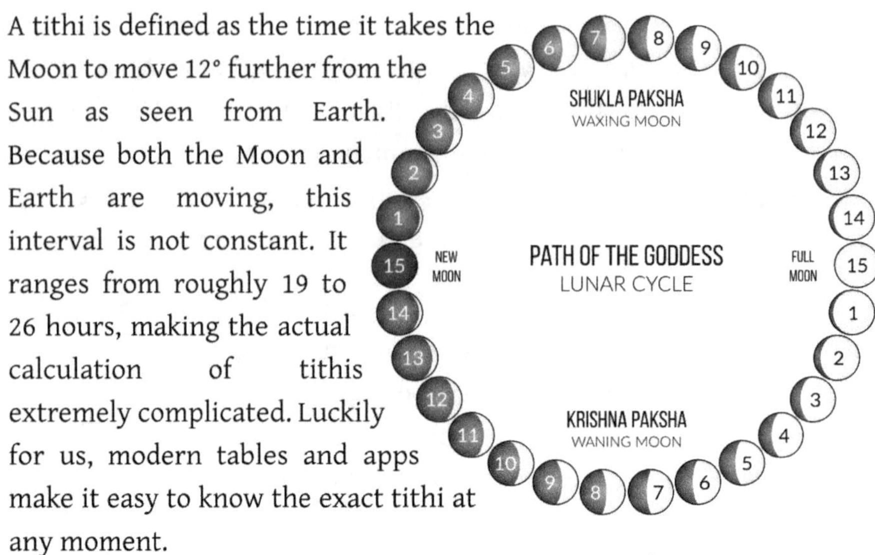

Each tithi carries its own energetic quality, and together with the horas, offer far more nuance than a simple Svara correspondence, which are taught within the greater meliu of tantric and astrological teachings,

In this publication I will limit myself to the instructions given in the Svara Śāstra, which give us a straightforward practical key: each lunar day (tithi) has a particular Svara that ideally should be active at sunrise and another at sunset, And when your personal Svara matches the natural Svara of the tithi, you are considered to be in alignment with nature.

Svara Flow in the Bright Fortnight (Śukla Pakṣa)

Let's start with the waxing moon, or bright fortnight. Svara Yoga gives a specific pattern for how the nostrils ideally flow at sunrise and sunset.

On the first lunar day (Pratipadā), the day after the new moon, the left nostril (Idā) should be active at sunrise and the right nostril (Piṅgalā) at sunset.

The sequence for Śukla Pakṣa is:

Tithis	Sunrise	Sunset
1–3 (Pratipadā–Tṛtiyā)	Left (Idā)	Right (Piṅgalā)
4–6 (Caturthī–Ṣaṣṭhī)	Right (Piṅgalā)	Left (Idā)
7–9 (Saptamī–Navamī)	Right (Piṅgalā)	Left (Idā)
10–12 (Daśamī–Dvādaśī)	Right (Piṅgalā)	Left (Idā)
13–15 (Trayodaśī–Purṇimā)	Left (Idā)	Right (Piṅgalā)

This means, for example, that if you wake on the first lunar day and find that your right nostril active at sunrise, you are out of alignment with the natural pattern. In that case, you can gently shift the breath to the left nostril to synchronize yourself with the tithi and its cosmic rhythm.

Svara Flow in the Dark Fortnight (Kṛṣṇa Pakṣa)

After the full moon, as the Moon wanes, the sequence reverses. In the dark fortnight, the ideal nostril dominance at sunrise and sunset follows this pattern:

Tithis	Sunrise	Sunset
1–3 (Pratipadā–Tṛtīyā)	Right (Piṅgalā)	Left (Idā)
4–6 (Caturthī–Ṣaṣṭhī)	Left (Idā)	Right (Piṅgalā)
7–9 (Saptamī–Navamī)	Right (Piṅgalā)	Left (Idā)
10–12 (Daśamī–Dvādaśī)	Left (Idā)	Right (Piṅgalā)
13–15 (Trayodaśī–Amāvasyā)	Right (Piṅgalā)	Left (Idā)

Again, these are not solar calendar days—these are lunar days, and a single solar day can sometimes contain two or even three tithis, so the lunar day may shift between sunrise and sunset. This is why anyone wishing to follow this practice accurately is encouraged to use a traditional almanac or a modern app that tracks the current tithi, then match the Svara accordingly.

The Yearly Cycle

Beyond the daily, weekly, and monthly cycles, Svara Yoga has a yearly one:

The six months of Uttarayana (Northward Journey): This is the six-month period of *Uttarayana*, when the sun appears to move north beginning at the Winter Solstice (around December 21st), is associated with Piṅgalā energy— activity, growth, and auspiciousness—as increasing daylight and growing warmth gradually lead to the Summer Solstice. In the Northern Hemisphere, this corresponds to winter, spring, and the beginning of summer.

The six months of Dakṣiṇāyana (Southward Journey): The following six months, *Dakṣiṇāyana*, begin at the Summer Solstice (around June 21st), when the sun appears to turn south. This half of the year aligns with the Idā energy—introspection, rest, and meditative qualities— as decreasing daylight and a gradual move towards coolness leads to the Winter Solstice, through late summer, autumn, and the beginning of winter. This division corresponds to the solar month cycle and influences seasonal and spiritual rhythms.

Aligning Yourself to Nature

One way to use this knowledge is to align with nature. When you are in harmony with nature, life tends to flow more smoothly, and when you are not, obstacles are more likely to appear— this is one of the key teachings of Svara Yoga.

Begin by checking your dominant nostril at sunrise. Ideally, it should correspond to the Svara indicated on the table for the current lunar day. If it does not, you can gently shift the breath to the correct side, and, in doing so, attune yourself with the tone of the day and subtly increase your likelihood of ease, support, and success in all your daily activities.

After aligning your nostril at sunrise, check again at sunset. If your svara still matches what the tithi table describes, you can assume that you have managed to return harmony with the natural cycle. If it has diverged, then something in the flow of your day has pulled you out of sync. For example, on the first day of the lunar month, the left nostril should be active at sunrise and the right at sunset. Waking with the left nostril active is ideal. But if, by sunset, the left nostril is still dominant and not the right, it suggests that you have drifted out of rhythm with nature and a gentle shift of the breath to the right nostril can help restore balance and support a deep, regenerative sleep.

You can also look into what, during the day, pulled you out of your center—what may have disrupted your connection with the natural field. In modern life, especially in a city, nature's rhythms are harder to feel. And it is completely natural to find yourself out of alignment from time to time.

When that happens, one of the simplest remedies is to literally reconnect with the living world: go outside into nature whenever possible, or bring a touch of nature indoors. Plants are far more sensitive than we are to the movement of the sun, so even if you cannot consciously sense these subtle shifts, the plant will—and you can, in turn, attune yourself to the plant.

If you find yourself out of alignment regularly, I suggest placing several plants in your home, especially species that feed directly on sunlight. Many diurnal or day-blooming plants open their flowers during the day and close them at night: African daisies, crocus, dandelion, evening primrose, gazania, kalanchoe, lotus, morning glory, poppy, sunflower, tulip, water lily, moss rose, and day-blooming cestrum are just a few examples. These flowers visibly respond to the sun's rhythm, unfolding with the daylight and folding again at dusk. Even if you are not consciously tracking it, your system will feel this rhythm, and over time it will coax your own nervous system back to a more natural flow.

Another powerful way to maintain harmony with the natural rhythm is through regular exposure to natural light. Most of us live and work in environments filled with artificial illumination, yet it is the subtly, continuous changes in daylight that give our bodies its cues for regulation.

The color and intensity of the sky vary throughout the day—between sunrise, midday, and sunset—and these subtle shifts signal the body when to awaken, when to act, and when to soften into rest. Working or practicing in a space with an open window or clear view of the sky helps the nervous system stay in tune with these cycles.

When you combine these two elements—aligning yourself breath with the appropriate svara each morning and remaining in touch with the natural light of day—the chances are much higher that, by evening, your breath, energy, and awareness will all be aligned with the rhythm of nature.

What Happens When You Are Out of Sync?

According to *Śiva Svarodaya*, when your breath consistently flows opposite to the Svara that should be active, negative effects begin to accumulate over time.

Verse 82 describes a progression of results if, morning after morning, the opposite Svara is flowing.

"If in the morning the opposite Svara flows, these are the results:

- 1st day – fickleness of mind,
- 2nd – loss of wealth,
- 3rd – unnecessary travel,
- 4th – destruction of cherished things,
- 5th – collapse of the home,
- 6th – loss of valuables,
- 7th – illness,
- 8th – death".

If this irregularity continues for many days, the text suggests that the results grow more severe—but it also assures us that even a small correction "brings fortune". In practical language, this means that even partial alignment helps, and that theSvara can serve as a daily diagnostic: it shows whether you are moving in harmony with nature or drifting away from it.

Combining the Systems

More than a tool for diagnosis, Svara yoga is a sophisticated science for finding the right moment for different kinds of actions. We have already seen how the text particular activities with either the left or the right svara (Chapter 8), and and how external cycles—yearly, monthly, weekly, and hourly—each carry their own energetic "breath".

So what do we do with all of this?

One possibility is to begin layering these systems— the yearly cycle, lunar cycles, planetary days, and hours—together so that your choices ride several supportive currents at once and you could pinpoint exceptionally auspicious moments.

For instance, imagine a Monday morning during the bright fortnight in September, at an hour that corresponds to the Moon. If you ensure that your Idā nāḍī is active and then choose a gentle, creative, or inward-oriented activity as described in Chapter 8, the tradition says that your chances of success are highly amplified.

Conversely, a Saturday during the dark fortnight in March, with your Piṅgalā active. That kind of moment would favor clear, decisive, or extroverted actions.

The more these cycles are brought into alignment —breath with body, body with day, day with season—the more your outer actions begin to resonate with the cosmic breath. Over time, Svara Yoga becomes less about controlling circumstances and more about learning to move when the universe is already exhaling in the direction you want to go.

The *Śiva Svarodaya* on Optimal Timing

The *Śiva Svarodaya* offers very concrete guidelines on timing.

Verse 69: "The actions done on Wednesday, Thursday, Friday, and Monday when the left Svara flows are most fruitful, especially during the bright fortnight".

In practice, this means that when your Idā nāḍīis active on these days—and you choose a gentle, creative, or inward-oriented action like those listed in Chapter 8—the tradition considers your chances of succeeding to be highly amplified.

Conversely, **Verse 70** teaches: "When the right Svara flows on Sunday, Tuesday, and Saturday, whatever business is done becomes most prosperous, especially during the dark fortnight".

These moments, combined with an active Piṅgalā, favor decisive, outgoing, or extroverted actions.

The essence of the teaching is this: if you have an important decision or undertaking before you—buying property, starting a business trip, making a major commitment—it is ideal to time it according to the appropriate hour, day, fortnight, season, and Svara combined.

In Closing

This chapter is admittedly quite technical, and perhaps can feel even overwhelming at first reading, like a lot to hold in mind all at once.

It also took quite some time for me to really understand how all these interlocking cycles—days, tithis, and Svaras—work, and become clear in lived experience.

So there is no need to rush. Don't worry if it feels complicated; that's because it is. But it's also profoundly beautiful once it "clicks".

I encourage you to go through it a few times, take notes, and, most importantly, experiment gently in daily life. Begin simply—perhaps just notice which planetary hour you're in during key moments of your day. Notice whether important communications tend to flow more smoothly during Mercury hours, or whether you feel naturally more energized and ready to move during Mars hours.

As you keep observing how your breath changes with the Moon and the days, it becomes clear that Svara Yoga is truly a science of cosmic synchronization. When the microcosm of your breath and the macrocosm of the universe begin to breathe together, life itself begins to flow with a different kind of ease and grace.

Chapter 15
How Long Is Your Breath?

After having learned how to identify which Svara is active in any given moment, and which kinds of actions are supported by each Svara, the tradition invites a closer look to another key feature of the breath: it's length. Observing the length of the breath reveals yet another layer of how prāṇa behaves as activities, times of day, and inner states change.

Understanding the Length of the Breath

In our context, the length of the breath is the distance from your body where you can still feel the breath. This might be where you can still feel the air on your skin or where it still produces a mark of condensation on a mirror.

You can explore this directly: cup one hand and place it gently underneath your nose. Breathe in and out naturally, without altering any aspect of your breath, then, slowly move your hand away from your nostrils, following the angle at which the air naturally flows, until you reach the point where you can no longer feel the breath hitting your palm.

It is important that you are not modulating your breath, breathing more strongly or softly—the enquiry works only when the breath is as unforced and ordinary as possible. You can even move your hand a little closer and farther to find the precise boundary where the touch of the breath fades.

Some practitioners use a mirror, watching for the tiny spots of condensation as they exhale. This can work, though it is less reliable since condensation depends on the humidity and temperature in the room, so the hand method is usually a better guide.

Once you've found the furthest point at which you clearly feel your breath, the yogis would traditionally measure the distance from that point back to your nose. The unit that the yogis used is called an *aṅgula*—one finger's breadth—this measurement, means it is always proportional to the person measuring, but roughly, on average it corresponds to between one and one and a half centimeters, or about half an inch. This simple measurement becomes the basis for understanding how the "reach" of the breath expands and contracts with different states of body and mind.

The Breath in Different Activities

Svara Yoga teaches that the length of the breath naturally changes with different activities and states. Some texts describe the natural length of the breath as seven *aṅgulas* (finger-breadths), while most texts give twelve *aṅgulas* as the usual distance.

During states of emotion and excitation, the breath can extend outward up to thirty-six *aṅgulas*. While singing it is said to be around sixteen *aṅgulas*; while vomiting, about eighteen. While eating, some texts say eighteen and others say twenty; while walking, the breath may extend up to twenty-four *aṅgulas*, and while running, to forty-two. During sleep, sources differ: some texts describe a length of thirty-six, while others claim it can reach one hundred *aṅgulas*. While copulating, some texts again mention thirty-six *aṅgulas,* while others give sixty-five.

The *Kālacakra Tantra* adds an important nuance: there is an inverse relationship between external and internal breath. The farther the breath extends outward from the nostrils, the less deeply it is said to penetrate within.

Thus from this viewpoint, a short, shallow external breath—one that stops close to the nose—actually indicates deeper internal penetration, reaching further into the core of the body and being. In other words, what looks small on the outside may be more powerful on the inside.

The yogis regarded each breath as a finite expression of life force, a precious resource to be used consciously and with intention. The more the breath was allowed to leave the body, to spill outward, the more it was believed that one's own vitality was being depleted, diminishing their health and even shortening their lifespan.

For this reason, the yogis recommend to shorten the length of the breath as much as possible, within what is natural for the activity at hand. A breath that is longer than the ranges mentioned above was considered a sign of disturbance or ill health, whereas a shorter (that is, externally shallower) breath appropriate to the situation was considered a sign of good health and balanced prāṇa.

Activity / State	Length (aṅgulas)	Comment
Natural at rest	7–12	Normal relaxed state
Singing	16	Controlled extended breath
Vomiting	18	Forceful exhalation
Eating	18–20	Moderate exertion
Walking	24	Moderate activity
Running	42	Vigorous activity
Sleeping	36–100	Slow metabolism
Copulating	36–65	Excited state

Modern Parallels

Modern medicine actually supports this traditional intuition about breath and vitality. The healthier and more conditioned the person is, the slower the resting heartbeat and the less oxygen is needed to sustain the same amount of activity, because . the cardiovascular system and lungs work more efficiently. This means the body can extract oxygen from the air more effectively and requires less at rest.

That's why athletes can have resting heartbeats so low that, in a sedentary person, would be flagged as unhealthy. The same goes for breathing: not just the number of breaths per minute, but the volume of air per breath, tends to be lower in those who are fitter, since their bodies extract oxygen more effectively.

From this perspective, the yogic connection between a "shallower" breath and robust health is indeed real: the healthier or more athletic the person, the less breath is needed to produce the same physiological effect.

The Breath and Meditation

Meditators also notice a similar pattern. As consciousness settles and deepens in practice, the breath often becomes subtler and externally shorter, sometimes to the point where it feels as though it almost disappears.

The *Śiva Svarodaya*, beginning in verse 224, teaches what happens when the breath naturally becomes shorter or shallower, and how such shortening is related to inner stillness rather than strain.

Measuring Your Own Breath

Because this teaching is meant to be experiential, I invite you to try it for yourself. Ssit comfortably and restfully, and begin by simply observing your natural breathing, without trying to deepen or soften it. Then, using the same method as before, cup your hand and place it beneath the nostrils. Breathe in and out in a relaxed, unforced way, and slowly move your hand away, following the natural angle of the exhaled air, until you locate the farthest point at which you can still feel the breath. These first steps call for a meditation like *Ānāpānasati*, simply observing the breath without trying to control it.

Once you've found the point, keep your hand there and use the other hand to measure in a simple, tactile way: Place the edge of your other hand at a right angle (90°) to the first hand, palm to palm, with the fingers outstretched and the thumb ignored. If you look at that side-view of the palm (without the thumb), you have four *aṅgula,* or finger-breadths.

Now slide the first hand—the one that was feeling the breath—up between that measuring hand and your nose, like forming an X-shape at the side of your face. Now you have eight *aṅgulas.* Continue like this hand-over-hand until you reach your nose. this gives you a measurement of how many finger-breadths the breath extends during a relaxed, neutral state.

According to the *Śiva Svarodaya*, an average, healthy breath at rest should extend to about twelve fingers away from the nose. If your breath is less than that distance, the *Śiva Svarodaya* would consider you healthier than average; if longer, you're either not at rest or there is room to improve your cardiovascular condition. To be clear, this method is not very accurate, so don't stress if you realize that your breath is a bit longer than the suggested 12 fingers.

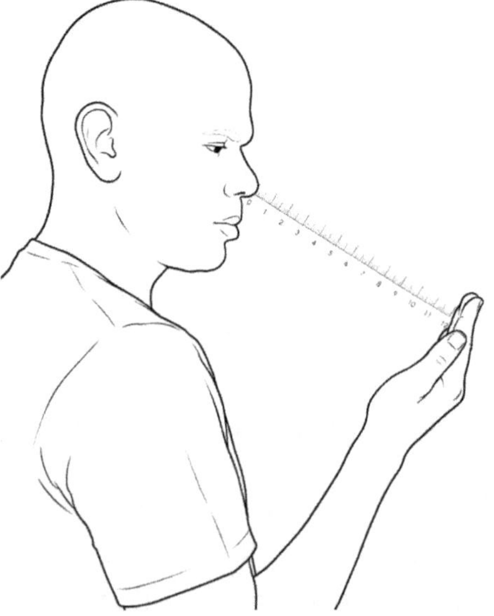

Progressive Shortening of the Breath

The *Śiva Svarodaya* next invites a direct, embodied exploration of what happens as the breath becomes shorter and shorter. To understand this, first measure out twelve fingers away from your nose, as a standard reference distance, regardless of your own breath length.

To do this, place the left hand so that the index finger lightly touches the nose and the pinky points at about a 45° angle, following the usual direction of the exhaled air.

Then place the index finger of the left hand onto the pinky of the right hand, keeping the right hand steady. Remove the left hand and bring it behind the right hand so that its index finger again touches the right pinky. Finally, lay the right palm flat on the pinky of the left hand.

At this point, your palm should be facing you at a distance of twelve fingers away from your nose. As you read through the subsequent verses in the text, you can slowly move your hand closer to your nose one aṅgula at a time to feel and visualize what it means, in Svara Yoga terms, for the breath to grow shorter and more refined.

Teachings from the *Śiva Svarodaya* (Verses 224 onwards)

> "If a yogi succeeds in reducing the length of prāṇa by one finger out of twelve, he obtains desirelessness.
>
> With a reduction of two fingers, he attains bliss
>
> If reduced by three fingers, he gains the energy of love.
>
> Now we are nine fingers away from the nose.
>
> Reduction by four fingers from twelve gives the power of speech—whatever is said comes true. This is known as *vāk-siddhi.*
>
> Reduction by five brings telepathy.
>
> By six, the ability to levitate.
>
> Reduction by eight fingers gives attainment of the eight siddhis. "

The Eight Siddhis

The yogic tradition describes eight primary *siddhis*—extraordinary capacities or paranormal powers— that can awaken as consciousness refines. These are often portrayed as expressions of a mind and body fully aligned with the subtle forces of reality.

- *Aṇimā* – the power to reduce the body to the size of an atom.
- *Mahimā* – the power to expand the body to an infinite size.
- *Garimā* – the ability to become infinitely heavy.
- *Laghimā* – the ability to become completely light.
- *Prāpti* – the ability to be anywhere at will.
- *Prākāmya* – the ability to obtain anything desired and realize whatever is wished.
- *Īśitva* – the power to create and control the forces of nature.
- *Vaśitva* – the power to bring all things under one's influence.

In many phases of yogic history, these siddhis wereseen as the highest goals, signs of becoming like Śiva himself—one radiant form of divine consciousness. Over time, many teachers began to emphasize that these capacities, while fascinating, are by-products rather than the true aim of practice, which is awakening to that consciousness itself.

Continuing with our text:

"Reduction by nine fingers gives the attainment of the nine *nidhis* or treasures, given to Hanumān, representing mastery over the universe".

"Reduction by ten gives the ability to change the body into ten forms (likely the ten forms of Viṣṇu)".

Now, just two finger-breadths from the nose, the breath must be so shallow—so subtle that you can barely feel it at that distance, and that even the smallest movement of the hand makes the sensation disappear.

"Reduction by eleven finger-breadths makes the body shadowless".

This state likely refers to the attainment of the *vajra-deha*—the "diamond body" or "light body", as described in the yogic and tantric traditions. As the *Praśna Upaniṣad* says:

"Prāṇa springs from the Ātman and is as inseparable from the Self as the shadow is from he who casts it".

Hence, when one has no shadow, one is no longer dependent on prāṇa. Prāṇa has no more control over such a being, who abides as pure *Puruṣa*, the Self.

"Finally, reduction by twelve finger-breadths enables one to attain the state of Haṃsa and drink the nectar of the Gaṅgā".

The teaching is pointing to a condition in which the breath has stopped completely. In other words, respiration as a physiological process has stopped, indicating complete transcendence of prāṇa's movement.

Reduction from 12 aṅgulas	Attainment / State	Sanskrit Term (if given)
1	Desirelessness	Vairāgya
2	Bliss	Ānanda
3	Energy of love	Prema-śakti
4	Power of speech (truthful speech)	Vāk-siddhi
5	Telepathy	—
6	Levitation	—
8	Eight siddhis	Aṇimā, Mahimā, Garimā, Laghimā, Prāpti, Prākāmya, Īśitva, Vaśitva
9	Nine treasures (HanumŌn)	Nava-nidhi
10	Ten forms of body (Viṣṇu)	Daśa-rūpa
11	Shadowless body	Vajra-deha
12	State of Haṃsa	Haṃsa-avasthā

The State of Haṃsa

According to the tradition, the yogi who mastered prāṇa from head to toe is said to become free from the need for food and has no desire to eat. The length of the breath is understood as directly correlating to the depth of consciousness: as awareness moves into the deepest states known as *samādhi*, the breath becomes so subtle that it could no longer be detected, this is the meaning of the "cessation of the twelve angula breath".

The yogis believed, at these depths, that the breath stopped completely and the practitioner entered a kind of stasis, no longer needing to drink, eat, or even age in the ordinary way. In my deep meditations I have experienced this total cessation of breathing, for what might have been five minutes or more. However, the perception of time in those moments is very different from normal. What seems like five minutes may be shorter, and the absence of sensation does not necessarily mean the body has ceased breathing. What is certain is that if the body continues to breathe, the breath is incredibly shallow and slow and imperceptible to awareness.

Subjectively, you can't feel yourself breathing. There is no sense of the lungs expand or the abdomen moving. The body feels utterly motionless. This profound stillness of body is coupled with a complete quiet of mind, and together they are described as the state of *Haṃsa*, where one "drinks the nectar of the Gaṅgā"— a poetic way of pointing to an inner current of bliss and luminous awareness

Symbolism of the Gaṅgā and the Nāḍīs

The Gaṅgā (*Ganges River*) is one of the most sacred rivers of India. Within Svara Yoga, references to Gaṅgā are often symbolic:

- *Gaṅgā* corresponds to the *Iḍā nāḍī*,
- *Yamunā* to the *Piṅgalā nāḍī*, and
- *Sarasvatī* to the *Suṣumṇā nāḍī*.

Their meeting point (*Triveṇī Saṅgam*) lies in the *Ājñā Cakra*. In this context, "drinking the nectar of Gaṅgā" represents absorption into the subtle current of *Iḍā nāḍī* and the experience of an almost immortal, cooling bliss.

Outside of Svara Yoga, Gaṅgā is also linked with the *amṛta*, the nectar of immortality. In mythology, Gaṅgā descends from the heavens as a goddess whose waters bring life and liberation, and even a drop of her water placed on one's lips at the moment of death is said to grant salvation (*mokṣa*).

Final Reflections

The text concludes this section by saying:

"Thus, the method of achieving all kinds of success through control of prāṇa has been described. This knowledge comes only through the Guru's instruction, and no amount of study can provide it".

Guru here means a living teacher, pointing to realization as something transmitted and embodied through direct practice, not just conceptually understood.

Now you know what to expect when meditating and your breath becomes progressively shallower and subtler, and how this process influences well-being, longevity, and the emergence of extraordinary states.

From here, the *Śiva Svarodaya* next introduces *prāṇāyāma* as the main technique to consciously control the breath and expand consciousness.

Chapter 16
The Most Essential Prāṇāyāma

I want to teach you one of the most fundamental *prāṇāyāmas* techniques in yoga, normally practiced within alternate-nostril breathing. Because there is no live guidance here to correct subtle mistakes, I will begin by teaching this practice as a straightforward *prāṇāyāma* with inhalation through both nostrils, making it less prone to mistakes that can actually imbalance you.

Precautions Before Practice

A word of caution: this type of *prāṇāyāma* is very deep, and can be harmful if done incorrectly, but only in the more advanced alternate-nostril form. It changes subtle aspects of our *prāṇa* as well as our consciousness, This version is gentle and safe, provided the following precautions are observed:

- You must have no cardiovascular illness or breathing problems.
- You must be in general good health.
- You must practice in a clean environment—clean in the physical sense of air quality, but also emotionally, mentally, and *prāṇically*.

If there is any doubt about suitability, seek the guidance of a qualified teacher who can personally assess and advise you. It is also important that both nostrils are open before you begin. If they are blocked, first perform *neti* (nasal cleansing) or the earlier techniques for modifying the svara on both sides to open the flow sufficiently for practice.

Preparation for Practice

Once both nostrils are open, you can begin. This *prāṇāyāma* does not depend on whether the active flow *(svara)* is on the left or the right. Sit in a comfortable position with your spine free and upright—either on the ground in any meditation posture or on a chair, making sure that your back does not lean against the backrest.

All breathing in this practice happens only through the nose, with both inhalation and exhalation nasal.

The Four Phases of Breath

According to yoga, our breath has four phases, and this technique is framed within that classical fourfold cycle:

1. **Inhalation** (*pūraka*),
2. **Internal retention** (*antar kumbhaka*), holding the air inside the lungs,
3. **Exhalation** (*recaka*),
4. **External retention** (*bāhya kumbhaka*), holding the air outside.

Most *prāṇāyāmas* use what is called *dīrgha prāṇāyāma*—the long breath—which has three parts to the inhalation:

- **Abdominal breathing** (*ādhāra śvāsa*): expanding the abdomen, filling the lower lungs.
- **Thoracic breathing**: expanding the chest forward, sideways, and upward, filling the middle lungs.
- **Clavicular breathing**: slightly lifting the shoulders, filling the upper lungs.

If this "complete yogic breath" is already familiar, you may apply it to this exercise. However, in the beginning stages it may be set aside, because combining all three segments with the specific rhythm of this *prāṇāyāma* can be challenging; at first, focus on the rhythm itself.

The 1:4:2:1 Rhythm

What makes this *prāṇāyāma* special is its ratio between the four phases of breath: inhalation, internal retention, exhalation, and external retention.

The rhythm is **1 : 4 : 2 : 1**, meaning:

- For each unit of inhalation,
- Hold the air in for four units,
- Exhale for two units,
- Hold the air out for one unit.

This is not a *prāṇāyāma* with fixed timing, but with a **fixed ratio** that can be multiplied to lengthen the cycles while preserving its inner harmony. Multiplying the ratio, it remains the same, each step stretching the same underlying pattern. For example:

- **multiplying it by 3 we get: 3 : 12 : 6 : 3** – inhaling for three seconds, holding for twelve, exhaling for six, and holding out for three.
- **multiplying it by 4 we get: 4 : 16 : 8 : 4** – inhaling for four seconds, holding for sixteen, exhaling for eight, and holding out for four.
- **multiplying it by 5 we get: 5 : 20 : 10 : 5** – inhaling for five seconds, holding for twenty, exhaling for ten, and holding out for five.

From my long experience of teaching this *prāṇāyāma* , the practical minimum is a multiplication of four. Three seconds of inhalation is quite borderline, barely allowing an inhalation, much less a quiet one, whereas four seconds seems just enough to complete a full performance without strain.

You may have learned to fill the lungs fully, from the abdomen up to the clavicles. But in this *prāṇāyāma*, especially at first, you deliberately do **not** fill the lungs completely, and that's fine. There's no need to push the air in. Instead, allow the inhalation to be slow and smooth, adding volume only as the system adapts.

As your practice deepens, you may progress to multiplications of six or more: at six you can comfortably fill the lungs, eight becomes noticeably stronger, and twelve or sixteen counts belong to a more advanced and powerful level of work.

For example:

- **6 : 24 : 12 : 6** is strong and balanced.
- **12 : 48 : 24 : 12** and **16 : 64 : 32 : 16** are advanced practices.

However, I recommend beginning with the **4 : 16 : 8 : 4** rhythm.

Progressing Through the Multiplications

If you feel stable at one ration and wish to increase the multiplication, do so gradually after a few days of practice. Move from **4 : 16 : 8 : 4** to **5 : 20 : 10 : 5**, and so on.

When practicing higher ratios, never jump straight into the longest inhalation. Instead, always warm up: you first work with a lower multiplication (for example 4), then 6, then 8, slowly lengthening the cycle within the same practice, so the body and mind open into the depth rather than being pushed into it.

One complete cycle consists of:

- Inhalation (*pūraka*),
- Internal retention (*antar kumbhaka*),
- Exhalation (*recaka*),
- External retention (*bāhya kumbhaka*).

After each round of the four phases, you may increase the duration if you feel steady but never change in the middle of a cycle. You must complete a full cycle before changing the multiplication of the rhythm. Begin with about five minutes per session, then gradually add time week by week until you comfortably reach 30 minutes or more.

What is the purpose of this *prāṇāyāma? The invitation is to approach this experience* without comparison, goals, or fixed expectations, so that the experience can become genuinely self-reliant and intimate. So rather than outlining the full significance of this technique in advance, as you become more familiar with the technique, you will discover for yourself how it refines the breath and quiets the mind. What I can tell you at this moment is that this rhythm aligns you with the rhythm of *prāṇa* itself., which is said to pulsate in this very way.

Chapter 17
The Flight of the Swan: The Breath as Haṃsa Meditation

One of the most recurring elements explained in *Svara Yoga* is that the simple act of breathing in and out forms a continuous, unspoken mantra, called *Ajapa Japa,* or the *Haṃsa Mantra.* This chapter introduces the most famous *Ajapa Japa* meditation, which is considered one of the most fundamental and important meditations in both the Indian tradition in general and *Svara Yoga* in particular.

The Breath as Mantra

Various Indian texts state that the natural movement of the air in and out of the body inherently creates a subtle sound. This sonic quality of the breath is said to create a mantra.

Some of what are considered the deepest teachings of the Indian tradition hold that the evolution of human consciousness is propelled not only by experience but also by the power of speech and *mantras* vibrating through us. According to these teachings the mantra created by the breath, in its incessant movement in and out, is that which drives human evolution.

According to most Indian texts, the average human breath naturally cycles in and out 21,600 times per day. As the air comes into the body, it is said to produce the sound **"haṃ"**, and as it leaves the body, it produces the sound **"sa"**.

Put together, each full cycle of respiration produces the sound "haṃ-sa".

The Symbolism of Haṃsa: The Swan and the Soul

In Sanskrit, *haṃsa* means "swan", a traditional symbol of the soul. Just like the breath connects our consciousness to the body—and when that breath stops, life stops and the soul leaves the body—the swan symbolizes that which moves between worlds, mediating between the individual and the universal. Thus the breath continuously repeats *haṃ-sa, haṃ-sa, haṃ-sa* meaning "soul, soul, soul", not only connecting the individual to the universal, constantly repeating a spiritual mantra.

This spontaneous, wordless recitation is known as *Ajapa Japa:* a natural form of meditation that unfolds simply by breathing, gently guiding the evolution of consciousness throughout a lifetime towards spirituality, a path to evolution that does not depend on external events.

And so one of the fundamental meditations within the Indian tradition is simply becoming aware of this *Ajapa Japa* — to become conscious of the mantra repetition that naturally occurs as the breath comes in and out of the body.

It is considered that by connecting with this automatic mantra repetition, we may strengthen the felt connection with our soul and allow our breath to carry our awareness from the individual self (*Jīvātman*) to the universal self (*Parabrahman*).

Haṃsa and So'ham – Two Forms of Ajapa Japa

Most lineages associate the inhalation with *haṃ* and the exhalation with *sa,* giving the continuous mantra *"haṃsa".* However, some lineages reverse this, connecting exhalation with *haṃ* and inhalation with *sa,* which creates the sound **"so'ham"** ("I am"), another legitimate but less common form of *Ajapa Japa,* but carrying a similar essence.

So'ham means "I am" or "I exist", where thehe "I" refers not to the personality but to pure consciousness itself. Thus, practicing *so'ham* meditation invites a steady recognition of "I am-ness".

Both *haṃsa* and *so'ham* are accepted forms of *Ajapa Japa* practice.

The simple Haṃsa Meditation

Now let us explore the simple *Haṃsa* meditation, a direct way to rest attention in the natural mantra of the breath.

Begin by sitting comfortably, either in a chair or on the ground. Soften your entire body, scanning for any chronic contractions and consciously releasing tensions left by the day.

Relax your hands. You may place them in any *mudrā* that feels natural, or simply rest them on your lap. One recommended *mudrā* for this meditation is as follows:

Place your left hand on your lap, palm upwards, place your right palm face down and then grab your **left thumb** with your entire right palm, as a child holds the finger of an adult. Then close the left fingers around the right hand, and let this rest in your lap.

Settling Into Awareness of the Breath

From this settled posture, bring your awareness to your breath.

For this meditation, inhale and exhale through the nose — even though the subtle sound of *haṃsa* is more naturally audible through the mouth.

Do not change anything: there is no effort to deepen, lengthen, or shape it. Simply become aware of the breath as it naturally enters and leaves the body.

Do not attempt to create anything, and do not prevent anything from happening. Simply observe the breath as it comes in and goes out, not forcing or blocking anything.

If you notice that you have become lost in thought, recognize that the moment you realize this is the moment you have returned to awareness of your breath.

Hearing the Sound of Haṃsa

Once the body and breath are relaxed, begin to notice that the breath creates a sound as it moves in and out. If you listen closely, the inhalation begins to reveal itself as "*haṃ*" and the exhalation as "*sa*", forming a continuous inner repetition of the mantra *haṃsa* with every cycle as you breathe.

Because the practice uses nasal breathing, this may be very subtle, almost imperceptible outwardly. Yet if you listen inwardly, you will hear *haṃsa* being repeated again and again.

Deepening Into the Meditation

As you deepen into this meditation, the experience of sound shifts from something physical to something and more and more internal. Feel as though your heart itself is silently repeating the mantra—*haṃsa, haṃsa*—with each breath.

Notice the movement of *haṃ* with every inhalation, drawing your awareness inward — from the infinite (*Parabrahman*) into your own heart.

Notice the sound *sa* accompanying the out-breath, as your consciousness expands outward, re-uniting with the infinite.

Visualizing the Flight of the Swan

Keep noticing this movement — the breath coming in with *ha*, drawing your consciousness inward into the body, and each exhalation with *sa*, letting your awareness expanding beyond the body's limits. You may feel the in-breath focusing at a point in the center of the chest and as it leaves, it dissolves into **infinity** — perhaps above the head or beyond the body.

Feel how this ongoing repetition of *haṃsa, haṃsa* connects you each moment to the world around you and with infinite consciousness.

You may even perceive an inner image of a **swan flying in and out of your body**, symbolizing how each breath links your individuality with universality.

Union of Breath and Soul

Notice the sound *haṃ* that your soul and breath make as the body naturally inhales, bringing life into the system, and the sound *sa* as your exhalation connects you back to the vastness of the universe.

Do not change the breath. Simply observe how the body and soul naturally flow in and out with the mantra *haṃsa.*

Maintaining Awareness Beyond Meditation

As you come out of this meditation, notice that the breath quietly continues its natural rhythm—and with it, the inner repetition of the mantra *haṃsa.*

Gently open your eyes while staying tuned to this subtle movement of the breath and the mantra flowing with it: *haṃsa, haṃsa* — "I am the Swan. I am the Soul".

Let this awareness accompany you as you go about your day.

And from time to time, whenever you happen to notice your breathing during the day, also notice the mantra *haṃsa, haṃsa* repeating within you, reconnecting you to your soul, your purpose, and your spirituality.

PART III: WORKING WITH THE ELEMENTS

Chapter 18
Introduction to the Tattvas

While Svara Yoga is primarily focused on the science of air flow through the nostrils and the appropriate actions to take when the air is flowing through either the left or the right nostril to achieve the best outcome, it teaches of yet another powerful cycle to align our actions even more profoundly with the flow of nature. This cycle is the flow of the five elements —the tattvas—throughout the day.

Ancient Concepts of the Elements

From ancient civilizations to modern times, human beings have sought to explain what the world is made of. Today, the physical world is understood to be made from atoms and subatomic particles, but across the ancient world—from Greece to India and China—scholars believed that the world was made of four or five elements: earth, water, air, fire, and space itself.

This fourfold or fivefold division of all matter was the cornerstone of philosophy, science, and medicine for millennia. However, ideas about the meaning of these elements differed greatly from one civilization to another, and even from one philosopher to the next.

Historians believe that as early as the eighth century BCE, Greek philosophers of the Archaic period began formulating theories of the four classical elements. We don't know exactly, but it is speculated that the fourfold division of nature into elements is far older, perhaps going back 12,000 years or even earlier.

One of humanity's oldest symbols, the swastika— and yes, this symbol is much more ancient than the horrors it was associated with in the 20th century—illustrates this fascination with the fourfold symbolism. The original swastika depicts four lines, which can represent four directions, four gods, four celestial objects, or four elements circling around a central point, and is at least 10,000 years old, indicating that the number four held deep meaning for these ancient cultures.

Some cultures that, as far as we know, developed independently from the Greeks also divided the world into four elements. The Ponkas, for example, a tribe of the Sun Nation, separated their camps into four quarters dedicated to the different directions of the sky and the elements of earth, wind (air), thunder (fire), and water.

In the Greek tradition, it seems that Plato was the first to use the term "element" in reference to air, fire, earth, and water. The ancient Greek word for elements, *stoichion*, meant "smallest division". The Greeks believed that these four elements were themselves unchanging, and that everything in the world was made from them, held together or pushed apart by forces of attraction and repulsion, which caused substances to appear to change. This view is surprisingly similar to how elements and molecules behave at the atomic level.

Aristotle related each of these four elements to two of four sensible qualities and presented this in a diagram of two squares, one inside the other, where fire was both hot and dry, air hot and wet, water cold and wet, and earth cold and dry.

He then added a fifth element, ether, as the quintessence of the other four, reasoning that since fire, earth, air, and water were earthly and corruptible, the stars, in which no changes were perceived, could not be made of any of the four elements but must be composed of a different, unchangeable, heavenly substance. Prior to Aristotle, aehter had been believed to be a form of fire.

To the ancient Greeks, the four elements described not only the physical manifestations of the material world but also essential qualities of human nature. For instance, the earth, solid and substantial, was associated with the physical and sensual aspects of life. Water, flowing and ever-changing, expressed emotion and empathy. Air, beyond simply the atmosphere and breath, signified the mind, intelligence and inspiration. And fire, meaning both the sun and flame, indicated both creative passion and destructive zeal.

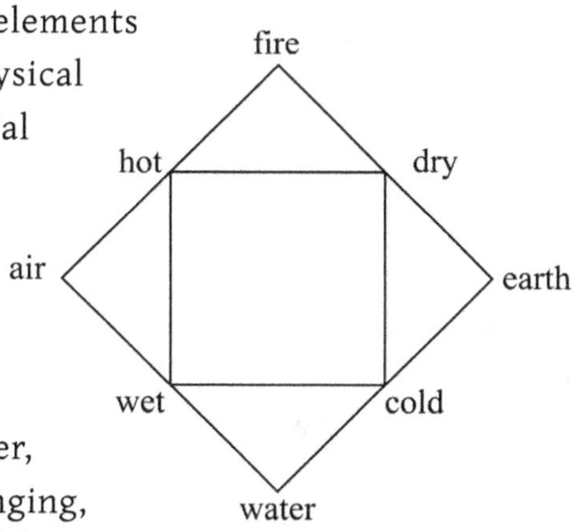

The Chinese and Indian traditions

The Chinese, on the other hand, developed a somewhat different series of elements during the Han Dynasty, around the first or second century BCE: wood, fire, earth, metal (literally gold), and water. However, these were understood as different types of energy or modes of transformation in constant interaction and flux with one another, rather than the different kinds of material substances as in the Western notion.

And so, these Chinese elements can't really be compared directly with the Greek elements, although they can, as we will see, relate quite closely to the *tattvas*, our subject of study within the Indian tradition.

Which brings us to the Indian and Buddhist traditions, both of which taught the existence of four great elements, called *mahābhūta*, said to comprise both the inner world of the body and the external world of objects: the earth element, *pṛthivī*; the water element, *āpas*; the fire element, *tejas*; and the air element, *vāyu*.

The earth element represents the quality of solidity or attractive forces. The water element represents the quality of liquidity or motion. The fire element represents the quality of heat, energy, and transformation. And the air element represented the quality of expansion or repulsive forces.

To these was added a fifth, physical element, the space element, *ākāśa*, corresponding to the Greek aether and representing the space in which all the other elements interplay. In time, a sixth element was added: consciousness, or *vijñāna*.

Tradition	Number of Elements	Elements	Nature of Elements	Key Idea / Function
Greek	4 + 1 (aether)	Earth, Water, Air, Fire, Aether	Material constituents	Four qualities: hot/cold, wet/dry
Chinese (Wu Xing)	5	Wood, Fire, Earth, Metal, Water	Energies / processes	Cycles of creation and destruction
Indian (Tattvas / Mahābhūtas)	5 + 1 (mind/ consciousness)	Earth (pṛthivī), Water (āpas), Fire (tejas), Air (vāyu), Ether (ākāśa), Consciousness (vijñāna)	Physical + psychological principles	Each linked to a sense, organ, and element of consciousness

Tattvas in the Indian Tradition

We will explore these more fully in the coming chapters and clarify how they connect to the subject of Svara Yoga. But before concluding this overview, I would like to note that these four, five, or six elements were not the final word. In fact, the Indian tradition continued this project of analyzing nature into building blocks, adding further principles beyond the mental element, eventually creating 25 separate *tattvas*, each representing another level or constituent of consciousness.

Although the *mahābhūtas* are already mentioned in the Vedas, it's in the Upaniṣads, around 800 BCE, that we first see a more systematic formulation of the *pañca mahābhūtas*—the five elements as such. Within the Indian tradition, each of the five elements was associated with specific senses, attributes, and functions within both the human being and nature, going far beyond the Greek conception of earth as roughness and solidity, water as liquidity, fire as heat, air as mobility, and *ākāśa* as space.

Each of the elements was associated with particular functions in the human body and in the natural world. The earth element, *pṛthivī*, was linked with odor and the sensation of smell, heaviness, steadiness, and material form. *Jala*, or water, with taste, coldness, and softness. *Agni*, or fire, with visible form or vision, brightness, digestion, and heat. *Vāyu*, or air, with tangibility and the sense of touch, roughness, emulsion, the structuring of body tissues, and the maintenance of movement within the body. Finally, *ākāśa*, the element of space, with sound and auditory sensation, as well as lightness, fineness, and space itself.

Each element was also assigned a mantra, a color (or *varṇa)*, and a *yantra*, a spiritual diagram. Together these associations allowed a rich meditative tradition centered on contemplating and working with the elements.

The elements in the body

The elements were also mapped onto the human being. The *Prapañca-sāra-tantra* explains that *ākāśa* is in the ears, *vāyu* skin, *agni* eyes, *āpas* tongue, and *pṛthivī* nostrils, corresponding to the organs through which we experience the senses connected with each *tattva*.

The *Śiva-svarodaya*, adds another layer, saying that fire is located in both shoulders, air at the root of the navel, earth in the region of the knees, water in the feet, and ether in the forehead.

In their subtler, spiritual form, the *tattvas* were placed along the spine, each one within a chakra: earth at *mūlādhāra* at the root, water at *svādhiṣṭhāna* in the pelvic area, fire at *maṇipūra* at the navel, air at *anāhata* in the chest, and *ākāśa* at *viśuddha* in the throat, with the sixth element of mind connected to the *ājñā* chakra, or third eye, in the middle of the forehead.

Each element was also said to be connected with a color: earth is yellow, water white, fire red, air blue or gray, and ether blackish or deep purple.

Each element was given a characteristic shape as well: earth a square, water a crescent moon, fire a triangle, air a hexagon or circle, and ether either a *bindu* (a dot), a downward-pointing triangle, or an overturned egg.

Regarding the mantras you may know them as "chakra mantras", but they are in fact mantras of the elements themselves: *laṃ* belongs to earth element, *vaṃ* to water, *raṃ* to fire, *yaṃ* to air, and *haṃ* to *ākāśa*, the ether element.

Each element was further connected with one of the subtle bodies: earth with the physical body, water with the pranic body, fire with the mental-emotional body, air with the wisdom body, and ether with the bliss body.

Each element also has a taste: earth is sweetish, water astringent, fire bitter, air acidic, and ether pungent and hot.

Tattva	Sense / Organ	Quality	Bija	Color	Shape	Chakra	Body	Taste
Earth	Smell / Nose	Solidity, stability	**Laṃ**	Yellow	Square	Mūlādhāra	Physical	Sweet
Water	Taste / Tongue	Fluidity, cohesion	**Vaṃ**	White	Crescent	Svādhiṣṭhāna	Prāṇic	Astringent
Fire	Sight / Eyes	Heat, transformat-ion	**Raṃ**	Red	Triangle	Maṇipūra	Mental	Bitter
Air	Touch / Skin	Movement, expansion	**Yaṃ**	Blue or Gray	Circle or Hexagon	Anāhata	Wisdom	Acidic
Ether	Sound / Ears	Space, lightness	**Haṃ**	Black / Deep purple	Downw-ard triangle or egg	Viśuddha	Bliss	Pungent

Application in Svara Yoga

For Svara Yoga, and for learning to recognize which action to take in which moment, the subject of the *tattvas* is of utmost importance. According to Svara Yoga, the *tattvas* flow through the universe in a specific cycle that manifests both in the external world and within our body, and each *tattva* has its own energy and its own vibration, making it auspicious or inauspicious for different kinds of actions.

If your actions carry the same quality as the *tattva* operating in that moment, then that moment is considered auspicious for those actions. And when the actions you want to take are not aligned—when they carry a different or conflicting energy or "vibe" than the *tattva* operating in the moment—then the moment is considered inauspicious, as if you are going against the flow. It's not the right moment. You need to catch the wave and wait until the vibration that suits your intended action has built up enough to carry you along with it.

In the following sections, we'll explore how the *tattvas* flow through the universe and the human being, how to identify which *tattva* is active at any given time, and which actions harmonize with each element.

Chapter 19
Alchemy Of Breath: Exploring the Elemental Shifts in the Svara

In this chapter, I want to focus on what Svara Yoga teaches about how the elements flow within human beings and within nature, one after the other, and which actions are recommended or should be avoided during each element.

The *Svara-śāstra*, the literature on *svara*, presents three distinct theories about how the elements, or *tattvas*, shift from one to another. The first theory is quite simple: it describes how the *tattvas* change in nature, independent of the human being who experiences them, so, we'll start here.

Theory One — The external cycle of the elements

According to this theory, the elements move through a cycle that begins at the moment of sunrise, when the ether element, *ākāśa*, rises. The cycles then moves from ether to air, from air to fire, from fire to water, and from water to earth, and once it reaches earth, the cycle restarts with earth shifting back to ether.

Each *tattva*, each element, is active for 24 minutes. So, starting at sunrise, ether rules for 24 minutes, followed by 24 minutes of air, then 24 minutes of fire, 24 minutes of water, and 24 minutes of earth, and then the pattern repeats with another 24 minutes of ether, and so on.

This cycle continues until the next sunrise. In a 24-hour day, we get 30 such shifts, But because the time of sunrise changes slightly from one day to another, the final *svara* of the cycle is often incomplete.

If sunrise occurs a little bit earlier than the previous day, the last *svara* will be slightly shorter—perhaps 23, 22, or 21 minutes, while if sunrise comes later, we'll have an "extra" *svara* during the night that might last only a minute, or perhaps five or ten, before ending at sunrise when the cycle resets itself and the ether element rules again for 24 minutes.

Now, we can make this picture a bit more complex. Within each *tattva*, the other *tattvas* also rise. This means that as the 24 minutes of ether begin, first it arises with the quality of ether within ether, followed by air within ether, then fire within ether, then water within ether, and finally earth within ether. Once this cycle within ether is complete, the pattern shifts into ether rising within air, then air within air, and so on.

This happens because each element reflects and contains the others. So even though ether is ruling those 24 entire minutes, we experience different modifications of the ether element: initially as pure ether, then as an airier expression of ether, and so forth, but it's still the ether element —100% ether— not the air element itself.

This level of detail is especially helpful when trying to pinpoint a very specific moment to support very important once-in-a-lifetime, or perhaps once-in-a-year event, because it has the potential to support the appropriate actions even more than just aligning them with the ruling element. But the difficulty is that within a 24-minute period, each tattva-within-tattva moment lasts less than five minutes and must be calculated with exact precision from the moment that the sun rises, which makes it a difficult calculation that most people struggle to get right.

For this reason, it's generally recommended to ignore this level of refinement unless we are very skilled in these calculations or have a highly accurate app to help us. What has been described so far is only the first type of cycle: it explains how the elements rise in nature around us, but not yet how they rise within us.

Order	Element	Sanskrit	Duration	Time after sunrise	Symbolic Phase
1	Ether	Ākāśa	24 min	0 – 24 min	Expansion / dawn
2	Air	Vāyu	24 min	24 – 48 min	Movement / change
3	Fire	Tejas	24 min	48 – 72 min	Energy / action
4	Water	Āpas	24 min	72 – 96 min	Adaptation / flow
5	Earth	Pṛthivī	24 min	96 – 120 min	Stability / grounding

30 cycles ≈ 24 hours.

Theory Two — The Internal Breath Cycle

The second and third theories describe how the *tattvas* arise within the breath itself: how they change the quality of the breath, and how, even within the lunar or solar *nāḍī* there are distinct types of breath that signals whether the fire, water, or earth *tattva* is active; how this changes the air flow within the nostril, and how we can sense which *svara* is active from within. The second theory is simpler to understand, so let's begin there.

According to this theory, within each *svara* the five elements rise one after another in the familiar order given, with each element occupying one *ghaṭikā* (24 minutes).

This means that when the breath starts to flow through the left nostril, from the moment it shifts, the breath first takes on the quality of ether, passing through a certain area in the nose with a distinct feel and temperature that persists for 24 minutes.

After these 24 minutes, the feeling of the breath—the area where it flows in the nostril, its path, texture, and temperature, shifts as the air *tattva* becomes active for another 24 minutes, followed by the fire element for 24 minutes, then water for 24 minutes, and finally earth manifests for 24 minutes.

Once the cycle of ether, air, fire, water, and earth is complete in one *svara*, the breath is said to shift to the opposite side. If the breath has been flowing in the left nostril, the breath shifts to the right, the solar *svara*, where it again begins with 24 minutes of ether, followed by 24 minutes each of air, fire, water, and earth, before shifting back to the lunar *nāḍī*.

Now, if these 24-minute segments, these *ghaṭikās*, are added up, this theory implies that the breath flows for two full hours in one nostril and then for two whole hours in the other nostril.

This second theory attempts to connect the external cycle described in Theory One with the way the same cycle manifests within us as individuals. But this doesn't sit comfortably with much of the rest of the Svara Yoga teachings, nor with what is known about the natural breathing cycles.

Svara Yoga sources mainly describe the breath cycle as being about 60 minutes long in each nostril. This is closer to what Western science observes: the nasal cycle can range between about 20 minutes and three and a half hours, with an average of roughly two and a half hours.

From this, we could argue that the yogis recommend aligning our breath so that the full cycle, left and right nostril, becomes exactly 120 minutes, with 60 minutes per side. But if we take the second theory literally, each nostril would need to flow for 120 minutes, making a full cycle about four-hours , something typically seen only with people who are ill.

In the text called the *Svara Cintāmaṇi*, we find the same theory, but with a different elemental order. Here, in the lunar *svara*, the *tattvas* are said to move from earth to water, fire, air, and finally ether—from the gross to the subtle—while in the solar *svara* the sequence is completely different: air, earth, water, fire, and ether. It's not clear why this order is given.

There's a strong possibility that this confusion arose during the process of creating and collating these texts. Looking at the *Śiva-svarodaya*, you'll see that it is very disorganized, which is often a sign that an author tried to weave together many small texts or conflicting source texts.

In places where such a synthesis was attempted, the result may be a kind of constructed theory that, when we examine it closely, loses its practical function and no longer fully makes sense.

Nostril	Element Order	Duration per Element	Total per Nostril	Total Full Cycle
Left (Lunar Svara)	Ether → Air → Fire → Water → Earth	5 × 24 min	120 min	≈ 4 h (in both)
Right (Solar Svara)	Ether → Air → Fire → Water → Earth	5 × 24 min	120 min	≈ 4 h (in both)
Variant - *Svara Cintāmaṇi*	**Left:** Earth → Water → Fire → Air → Ether **Right:** Air → Earth → Water → Fire → Ether	24 min each	120 min	≈ 4 h

Theory Three — Elemental Proportions within the Hour

The third theory, found in the *Śiva-svarodaya*, states that during the flow of a single *svara*, the elements arise in this order: air, fire, earth, water, and ether. All five appear during a period of two and a half *ghaṭikās*, or one hour.

The *Śiva-svarodaya* further explains that each *tattva* occupies a different proportion of that hour: earth is 50 parts, water 40, fire 30, air 20, and ether 10. Translated into a 60-minute cycle, this gives approximately 8 minutes of air, 12 minutes of fire, 20 minutes of earth, 16 minutes of water, and 4 minutes of ether.

at the end of this sequence, it is through the brief ether phase that the breath disperses and shifts into the other nostril, the other *svara*, where the cycle begins again with the air element.

A Fourth Theory from Vedic Astrology

Before closing, I want to mention one more related theory, not from the *svara* literature, but from Vedic astrology. This model also assigns different durations to the *tattvas*, but here the total cycle is 90 minutes long:

Earth dominates for 6 minutes, water for 12, fire for 18, air for 24, and ether for 30.

The elements are said to follow two possible orders:

1. Earth → Water → Fire → Air → Ether
2. Ether → Air → Fire → Water → Earth

According to this astrological view, each day of the week also begins with a different ruling *tattva*: Sunday with fire, Monday water, Tuesday fire, Wednesday earth, Thursday ether, Friday water, and Saturday air.

These timing schemes correspond to the planets and arise from Vedic astrological calculations. This theory is most often used to correct the recorded time of birth of an individual when the exact time is not known, helping to make more accurate astrological predictions.

Conclusion: Toward Direct Perception

I recognize that when hearing all these theories together, you may feel a bit confused and wonder, "So, which am I actually supposed to follow?"

Especially since in the next chapter, I'll teach you practical techniques that allow you to directly identify which *tattva* is active within you, so you won't need to rely on any theoretical model.

But by having these theories in the background, you'll be able to observe which external pattern your own internal rhythm is aligning with, or if it is not aligning with any at all, a possible sign of internal imbalance. Otherwise, in day-to-day life, most people tend to follow the first theory, simply because it's the easiest to apply.

Chapter 20
Tattva Vicāra: Direct Perception of the Elements

In this chapter, I want to focus on a few processes that teach us how to identify which *svara* is active at the very moment of observation. Some of these processes are internal, and some are external.

Tattva Vicāra – Inquiry into the elements

Let's start with a process called *tattva vicāra*, the inquiry into the *tattvas*. This method allows for the identification of the active *tattva* simply by feeling how the air flows inside our nose.

Each *tattva* causes the air to flow through different areas inside the nostrils, exit from slightly different points, and extend outward in different directions and distances from the body. Each *tattva* also has a slightly different quality of heat, dryness, or moisture, as well as other subtle characteristics which, if we take them together, make it possible to identify which *tattva* is currently active within us.

Characteristics of the Five Tattvas

Earth Element (Pṛthivī) - Air flows through the center of the nostril in a concentrated stream and exits straight forward, in line with the nostril's angle, reaching a distance of about 12 fingers. The breath is slow and slightly warm, making a deep sound while a sweetish flavor may be present in the saliva.

Water Element (Āpas) - Breath flows slightly downward, leaving the nostrils from the lower point close to the upper lip, and travels to a distance of about 16 fingers. The air is very fast, loud, and cold, and an astringent taste may be experienced.

Fire Element (Tejas) - The air is heated and flows upward, exiting from the point closest to the tip of the nose and extending upward for about 4 fingers, and feeling very hot. A bitter taste may accompany the breath.

Air Element (Vāyu) - Breath flows along the outer parts of the nostrils at a slanting angle, slanting left from the left nostril and right from the right nostril, reaching about 8 fingers. It's described as slightly cold, or alternating between cold and warm, and a sour taste may be present in the mouth.

Space Element (Ākāśa) - Air flow is evenly dispersed within the nostril and may feel as if it is not actually leaving the nose, yet it can be felt up to 20 fingers away. This is experienced as a mixture of all the elements. A pungent and hot taste may be perceived in the mouth.

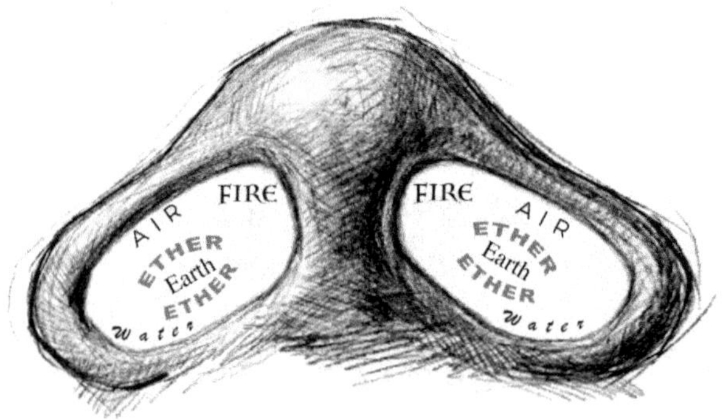

Practicing Observation

To begin exploring these sensations, find a comfortable seated position with your spine upright. Allow the breath to move in and out naturally through the nostrils without attempting to control or shape it.

Observe the breath gently. At first, it may be difficult not to unconsciously modify it. Often, for most of us, when beginning breath-awareness practices, we tend to modify the breath—making it deeper or shallower than usual or slowing it down. My invitation to you is to simply observe and let the breath be exactly as it is.

Start by noticing where the sensation of the breath is most pronounced in your nostrils:

- If it is strongest at the tip of the nose, the fire element is most likely active. But don't jump to immediate conclusions. Keep feeling and combine this sensation with all the other characteristics of the breath before deciding which *tattva* is present.
- If you feel the air close to the upper lip—the part of the nostril that is closest to your face, called the lower part of the nostril— this means that the water element is most likely active.
- If the breath flows mainly along the outer rim of the nostrils to the right and left, so that the sensations are strongest on the outer parts of your nostrils, this indicates that the air element is active.
- If you don't clearly feel the air passing inside the nostrils, either because it flows through the center or seems evenly distributed throughout, this may mean that the earth or ether elements are active. These two can be a bit confusing and require a closer inspection: if ti is the earth you will not feel the air at all as it passes through the center, if on the other hand you feel the air filling the entire nostril, touching and generating sensation on all its inner surfaces equally as it flows, you are likely sensing the ether instead.

Next, focus on the temperature of the breath:

- A hot or sharp sensation corresponds to the fire element.
- Cold air near the upper lip suggests the water element.
- Slightly warm or cool air on the outer rims of the nostrils may indicate the air element.
- A diffuse, warm sensation without a clear direction could reflect either ether or earth.

You can sense these temperatures inside the nostrils or, if you want, by holding your hand in front of your nose and feeling the air as it touches the skin.

You may also observe the direction in which the breath flows, either as a sensation inside the nostril or as it brushes along different areas of your face or body. Keep your hand about three inches away from your face to simply feel which part of the palm receives the air. Identify the direction as one of the following:

- If the air moves upward toward the eyes, this suggests the fire element.
- If it moves downward along the chest, this is likely water.
- If it goes straight forward, this implies earth.
- If the breath slants outward to the left or right, this points to air.
- Ether often feels like warmth without a distinct sense of motion.

Next, examine how far from the body the breath can be felt. Hold your hand next to your nostril, starting about two fingers away, and slowly move the hand farther until you can no longer feel the airflow, without changing your breathing, only change the position of your hand. Once you find the point at which the movement of air is no longer felt, measure that distance to your nostril. The general rules indicate that 4 fingers correspond to fire, 8 to air, 12 to earth, 16 to water, and 20 fingers, or a very diffuse sensation, to ether.

Finally, bring your attention to the taste in your mouth:

- Sweetish = earth
- Astringent = water
- Bitter = fire
- Acidic = air
- Pungent and hot = ether

Putting It All Together

Now that you've gathered these observations, reflect on which qualities seem to align.

Was the breath central, frictionless, slow, warm, straight, sweetish in taste, and reaching about 12 fingerbreadths in front of the nose? If many signs, like these, point towards the same *svara*, as they do to the earth element, it is most likely that you have figure it out. On the other hand if the signs are conflicting, then avoid jumping to any conclusions and simply give it a moment and test again; discerning the *tattva* is a very subtle process and it is possible that you are experiencing the shift of the element dominant in your breath.

A few more aligned examples will help us to clarify:

- If the air flows low and cold, downward and quickly, with an astringent taste, making a sound as it flows along your chest to a distance of about 16 fingerbreadths, this is likely the water element.
- Is your breath sharp, hot, upward-moving, short in reach, and bitter, extending upward to about 4 fingerbreadths? That would indicate fire.
- Is your breath slanted to the side from the outer part of the nostril, reaches a moderate distance of about 8 fingerbreadths, and feels cool or sour? These signs aligns with air.

- Does it feel more dissipated, with a soft warmth expanding in all directions and having a pungent quality? This most likely indicates the ether tattva.

If you didn't clearly feel any of this, I invite you to repeat this meditation several times. It takes a while to become familiar with these patterns of the breath.

I invite you, while doing silent meditation or breath-awareness practice, to gently bring this inquiry into the experience. This way, each session of breath meditation—every *vipassanā*, every *ānāpānasati*—becomes an opportunity to identify not only which *svara* is active, but also which *tattva* is active in every moment.

By practicing this way over a few days, weeks, or months, your sensitivity to these sensations grows, and recognition of the *tattvas* becomes much clearer.

An added benefit is that this kind of mindful observation helps to regulate the cycle of *tattvas* itself: if your cycle has become irregular or chaotic, sustained awareness of how the air is flowing in each and every moment gradually encourages the *tattvas* to align to one another and fall back into a more harmonious sequence.

The Mirror Technique

Finally, external paraphernalia can also be used to determine which tattva is active. Recall one of the first chapters in this book, where I taught you a technique to identify the active nostril by holding a mirror or other reflective surface underneath your nose and observing which side had the more prominent condensation.

In this chapter, I want to teach you to refine this same method to identify the active *tattva* by identifying the *shape* of the condensation on the mirror. According to the *Svara-śāstra*, each element has a distinct geometric shape associated with it, and this can be seen in the condensation patterns formed by the breath when that *tattva* is active.

The technique is simple. Sit comfortably and hold a mirror, smartphone or any smooth cold surface close to your nostrils, about four fingers away, just enough to clearly capture the condensation pattern.

The colder the surface, the longer the condensation will remain. However, if it's much colder than the surrounding air, it will begin to attract moisture from the environment, so it is best to practice in a relatively cool space with a slightly cool object.

Simply observe your breath without trying to modify or alter it. As you inhale, bring the mirror into position and allow the exhalation to flow naturally out of the nostrils, then lift the mirror and look at the shape that has formed.

The Five Elemental Shapes

- If the condensation forms a square, the Earth element (Pṛthvī-tattva) is active.
- If it appears as a crescent or half-moon, it is the Water element (Āpas-tattva).
- If the shape forms a triangle, the Fire element (Agni-tattva) is active.
- If it appears as a circle, the Air element (Vāyu-tattva) is active.
- And if the condensation has no defined shape or appears as scattered speckles, the Space element (Ākāśa-tattva) is active.

You can also note where on the mirror the shape appears, since each *tattva* directs the air flows differently.

- From the top of the nostril, making the condensation appear in the upper part of the surface, it is the Fire element.
- From the bottom of the nostril, causing the condensation to form in the lower part of the surface is the Water element.
- From the side of the nostril, the Air element, creates condensation on the sides
- And from the center of the nostril, the Earth and Ether elements forming condensation in the center

Look carefully at the mirror to see where the pattern is located. It may take several attempts, and even a few days of practice, before you can clearly identify the shapes and their subtle differences.

Finally, you can combine this mirror observation with the cues given in previous chapters by feeling the air inside your nostrils and noting which part of the nostril generates the most friction or sensation, the warmth or coolness of the breath, the taste in your mouth, the direction of the airflow, the distance it travels, and, finally, the shape of the condensation.

Chapter 21
Śanmukhī Mudrā:
Unveiling the Inner Vision of the Tattvas

In this chapter, we will explore the last of the techniques I will give for recognizing which *tattva* is active in the present moment, and in the following chapter, we will explore the actions that are recommended or that should be avoided in relation to each *tattva.*

The practice presented in this chapter is called **Śanmukhī Mudrā**, and through it you will learn to create an internal space in which the shape and color of the predominant *tattva* can appear in your inner vision. *Śan* means "six", and *mukhī* means either "faces" or "gates". and this is the technique that closes the six gates of the head, the six orifices of perception. By closing these we can create a state of withdrawal from the external senses opening us to observe subtle internal signs.

Performing Śanmukhī Mudrā

Sit in a comfortable meditation posture, this may be a simple cross-legged posture such as *Siddhāsana* or *Arda Siddhāsana*, but any meditation posture that you know will do, even sitting on a chair, as long as the spine is upright and relaxed.

Then, raise the elbows to the sides of the body and begin closing the "doors" of perception: Use the thumbs to gently close the ears, blocking external sound, the index fingers placed softly over closed eyelids, with only very light pressure blocks external light. The middle fingers close the nostrils blocking smell, and the ring fingers resting on the upper lip, with the little fingers on the lower lip block the sense of taste.

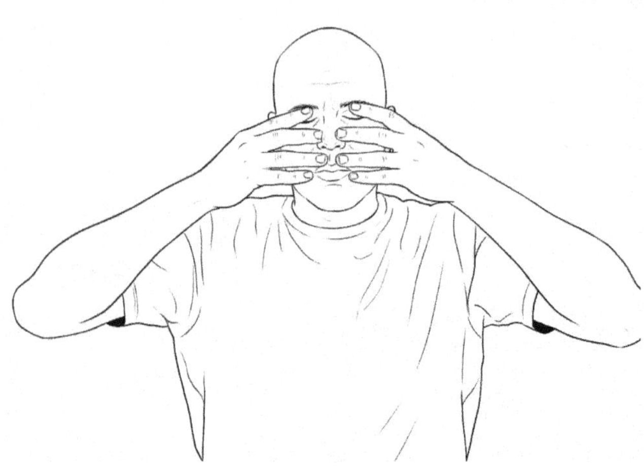

With the external senses blocked, the internal senses sharpen making the visions you are about to witness more vivid.

The Space of Awareness: Cidākāśa

This inner space, called Cidākāśa, is located roughly twenty centimeters in front of your forehead and extends upward about an arm's length toward the sky.

This is the recommended field for inner visualization, the subtle space where the *mind-stuff* (*citta*) projects its shapes and colors, like an internal screen on which the imagination unfolds. By softly gazing into this dark inner space behind the closed eyelids, colors and shapes may begin to arise.

These colors and shapes are said to correspond to the tattvas in the following manner:

- Yellow color or a yellow square – Earth (*Pṛthvī-tattva*)
- White color or a white crescent moon – Water (*Āpas-tattva*)
- Red color or a red triangle – Fire (*Agni-tattva*)
- Blue (sky-blue) or grayish color, especially forming a hexagonal star – Air (*Vāyu-tattva*)
- Complete darkness or shifting multicolored hues – Space (*Ākāśa-tattva*)

The last sign, space, corresponds to the *Ākāśa-tattva* only in the deeper stages of practice. At the beginning, it may simply indicate that the colors have not yet fully manifested.

Variations in Breathing

Different traditions describe several variations of *prāṇāyāma* to accompany this practice to aid in the intensification of the shapes and colors.

1. Inhale through the mouth in *Kākī Mudrā* (the "crow's beak") and exhale through the nostrils.
2. Inhale and exhale through both nostrils to activate the *tattva* and make the colors more vivid.
3. Inhale and exhale only through the active svara, if the lunar *svara* is active, use the left nostril; if the solar is active, use the right.

And so the technique proceeds as follows:

Start by exhaling all the air, emptying the lungs completely, and then, without pausing, inhale fully, filling the lungs entirely. You can perform a full yogic breath filling your lungs in a sequence from the abdomen, through the thorax and clavicular regions of the lungs. Or, you can just inhale normally without attention to a specific order.

Once your lungs are full of air, and without exhaling apply the *Śanmukhī Mudrā,* closing the gateways, and hold the breath as long as you can, gazing behind closed eyelids with both the physical eyes and the inner attention into Cidākāśa .

With *Śanmukhī Mudrā,* all the sense gateways are closed. The remaining two or three orifices in our body (depending on our biological sex) can also be gently "locked" with the *mūla-bandha*, *Aśvinī-mudrā*, and *Vajrolī-mudrā*, which basically means contracting all the muscles in the pelvic region, as if holding back the urge to urinate and defecate.

And then we simply observe. It may take several repetitions before shapes or colors begin to appear.

It is generally advised to begin with three to five repetitions and gradually increase to ten cycles.

You will usually notice the colors while the lungs are full. To complete one round, exhale the air completely at the end.

With consistent daily practice, once or twice per day, the ability to perceive these colors may develop over weeks or months, though for some practitioners it can arise even during the first session.

Initially, the colors might not be very distinct or clearly shaped, and the elements can appear mixed. One predominance does not exclude the presence of others, and this is perfectly fine. Don't worry if the colors seem blended at first. Over time, one will usually become more prominent and make itself known.

Chapter 22
What to Do on Each of the Tattvas

Now that you know it's possible to identify which *tattva* is active at any given moment, either through direct observation or by consulting *tattva* timetables, the next step is to understand which actions are considered auspicious or inauspicious during each element and to align activities with the natural rhythms of these elements.

The Earth Element (*Pṛthivī-tattva*)

When the Earth element is predominant, it is recommended to undertake stable and long-lasting deeds. This is an ideal time for construction—building a fort, house, mansion, city, village, or garden—as well as for defensive or stabilizing activities, even in the midst of conflict.

The *Śiva Svarodaya* states that Earth and Water bring accomplishment, so actions begun under the Earth *tattva* tend to yield enduring, steady results. The Earth element signifies solidity, longevity, and material prosperity.

The Water Element (*Āpas-tattva*)

When the Water element is active, it favors ceremonies and undertakings involving movement or union. This includes marriages, auspicious functions, travel, coronations, creating wells, ponds, or tanks, building or entering houses, journeys, sowing seeds, installing images of deities, performing *yajñas*, and intimate relations.

The *Āpas-tattva* signifies flow, adaptability, and fertility. Its results tend to be quick and fruitful, though somewhat more transient than those of the Earth element, making it well-suited to endeavors requiring flexibility, creativity, and connection.

The Fire Element (*Agni-tattva*)

The *Śiva Svarodaya* cautions that when the Fire element is active, harm or even death may occur. This *tattva* is therefore inauspicious for most actions, except those involving conflict, competition, intense tapas, or great exertion.

Fire burns and destroys what is unstable or premature, yet controlled fire can serve acts that require courage, purification, or decisive energy. During this time, it is wise to avoid impulsive speech, confrontation, or initiating new plans, as accidents, injuries, and heated arguments are more likely when *Agni-tattva* predominates.

The Air Element (*Vāyu-tattva*)

According to the *Śiva Svarodaya*, actions performed under the Air element tend to bring destruction or instability. The *Svara-cintāmaṇi* adds that during the *Vāyu-tattva* one may undertake deeds involving movement—such as mounting a horse, driving vehicles, or riding animals—yet it warns that this is an inauspicious time for marriage, travel, or warfare, as it may result in sickness, loss, or even death.

Air represents motion without clear direction, so actions initiated under this *tattva* can disperse energy without producing concrete, lasting results. Metaphorically, Air scatters rather than stabilizes, making it a time to ground, center, and refrain from starting important undertakings.

The Ether Element (*Ākāśa-tattva*)

No worldly work should be initiated while the Ether element predominates. As the *Śiva Svarodaya* says, everything tends to "draw to a blank" during this period.

The *Svara-cintāmaṇi* notes that although ordinary gain or loss usually does not occur in *Ākāśa-tattva*, for yogis it is a highly favorable time for meditation and spiritual practice. When Ether dominates, the mind naturally turns inward and becomes spacious, opening access to silence, intuition, and deeper awareness.

Summary of the Five Tattvas

Tattva	**Nature**	**Recommended Actions**	**Avoid**
Pṛthivī (Earth)	Stable, material, long-lasting	Building, steady work, financial or physical investments	Rapid change or travel
Āpas (Water)	Fluid, fertile, connective	Ceremonies, relationships, travel, creative work	Excess rigidity
Agni (Fire)	Transformative, volatile	Acts requiring courage or purification	Starting new plans, conflicts
Vāyu (Air)	Erratic, unstable	Movement, change (with caution)	Important decisions, commitments
Ākāśa (Ether)	Subtle, expansive, spiritual	Meditation, contemplation	Material pursuits

Additional Correspondences: Food and the Tattvas

The *Svara-cintāmaṇi* also assigns specific foods to each *tattva*: earth is linked with rice, sweet porridge, and tubers; water with oil and liquid meals; fire with flour, ghee, and oily preparations; air with greens and leafy vegetables; and ether with flowers. These recommendations attune the body to the energetic quality of the prevailing *tattva*.

Common Questions

What if an action takes longer than one Tattva?

Usually, what matters most is the moment of initiation. If an activity begins under an auspicious *tattva* (Earth or Water) it carries that energetic imprint even if it continues into less favorable periods. For instance, if a conversation begins under *Āpas-tattva* and passes into *Agni-tattva*, it may be wise to pause when the energy becomes heated, perhaps by taking a natural break if the other person is unfamiliar with the *tattvas*.

How do the Tattvas connect with the Svaras?

In general, *Pṛthivī* and *Āpas* (Earth and Water) are considered auspicious regardless of which *svara* is active. *Agni* and *Vāyu* (Fire and Air) may produce moderate results when they coincide with the lunar svara (left nostril) but tend to be especially disruptive under the solar svara (right nostril), while *Ākāśa* is ideal for meditation and is best practiced when the Sushumnā svara is active and the breath flows evenly through both nostrils.

Practical Application

There are two primary ways to apply this knowledge in daily life:

1. Internal observation: Determine which *tattva* is currently active within your body by observing your *svara* and the associated elemental qualities.
2. External calculation: Use astrological or time-based methods to determine which *tattva* is active in your environment.

With this understanding, your actions can be aligned as follows: Begin important ventures during Earth or Water *tattvas*. Choose Fire for physical, demanding, or competitive activities. Use Air for communication or light interaction, but not for making commitments. Reserve Ether for meditation and spiritual practice.

Now, equipped with the knowledge of *tattvas*, it becomes possible for you to consciously choose the right moment to begin any action, and as life is brought into harmony with these elemental rhythms, life's actions begin to align more naturally with success, ease, and balance.

Chapter 23
Elemental Trāṭaka: Harnessing Elemental Energy Through Gaze

Having now explored the elements in depth, I want to teach you one more technique to help you connect with them more directly. This practice is especially helpful if *Śanmukhī Mudrā* has felt challenging, particularly when it comes to perceiving the colors and shapes of the elements.

Before going into the technique itself, however, I want to share something about my teaching approach behind it. This will clarify why I don't recommend starting with this method immediately, but instead to give yourself a few weeks or even a few months of *Śanmukhī Mudrā* practice first.

My guiding principle between practice and theory is simple: *we practice first and explain later*. I know that many yoga schools follow a different approach, emphasizing the opposite order: "Here is the practice, here is what to expect, now let's practice it", but this tends to create expectations, and that can be a problem.

The Problem with Expectation

As both a student and teacher, I discovered that when I know beforehand what I'm "supposed" to experience, that knowledge colors the experience itself. With prior expectations it becomes difficult to distinguish whether something is truly being perceived in nature or whether my mind creates it in order to fulfill that expectation, a phenomenon psychology describes as being "primed" to experience it.

That is why, for me, it's very important to keep a *clean practice*, so that the genuine effects of our efforts can be observed without unnecessary mental interference. Hence, the "practice first, explain later" order.

Of course, this kind of purity is harder to maintain in an online platform or book, where you can read ahead. If we were working together in person, I would simply give one practice at a time. But in this format, my suggestion is: practice first, then seek understanding.

Now, I also want to clarify that providing theory before practice is not "wrong". In *Trika Śaivism* (Kashmir Śaivism), for example, it is posited that one can even *imagine* the results, and in time they will manifest. Tibetan Buddhism applies similar principles. So, this theory-first approach is entirely legitimate in spirituality. But my personal preference here is simply to emphasize direct experiences first and add the interpretive layer afterward.

Therefore, I recommend staying with the *Tattva-vicāra* and *Śanmukhī Mudrā* for some time before proceeding to this new method: the practice of *Trāṭaka* on the shapes of the elements.

What Is Trāṭaka?

Trāṭaka is a traditional *Haṭha Yoga* technique of steady, blinkless gazing on a single object.

When our gaze rests unmoving on a single object, the mind begins to merge with that object, thoughts are absorbed into it, and the mind begins to take on its qualities. This state of deep identification is known as *Saṃyama*, a meditative absorption in which the boundary between observer and observed dissolves. If the chosen object is water, for instance, the mind begins to *feel* watery—fluid, receptive, and reflective—illustrating how yogic insight into the elemental forces of nature is cultivated.

The yogis observed that eye movement is closely linked to thought movement: when the eyes are stilled, without blinking or shifting, the stream of thoughts also quiets. Staring at a blank wall can evoke the experience of *śūnyatā*, or emptiness, as is done in the *zazen* meditation in Zen Buddhism, whereas gazing at a bowl of water as done in the Buddhist *Kasiṇa* meditations attunes awareness to the consciousness of water itself.

The Practice of Elemental Trāṭaka

In this practice, we perform *Trāṭaka* on the visual symbols of the five elements.

Sit in a comfortable meditative posture, *Vajrāsana* (sitting on the knees, as in Zen) is ideal, and face a wall at about arm's length, just far enough that your fingertips can barely touch it when the arm is extended.

Place a diagram of the chosen element on the wall at about the height of your forehead so that your gaze is slightly lifted, and work with only one symbol per session.

The elemental symbols are as follows:

- Earth (*Pṛthvī-tattva*): a clay-yellow square printed on a white or black background.
- Water (*Āpas-tattva*): a white crescent moon resting on its side, placed on a black background.

- Fire (*Agni-tattva*): a red upward-pointing triangle.
- Air (*Vāyu-tattva*): a sky-blue circle or a smoky-blue six-pointed star (*Śaṭkoṇa*).
- Ether (*Ākāśa-tattva*): a downward-pointing black triangle or an egg-shaped form with purple or white specks, resembling stars in deep space.

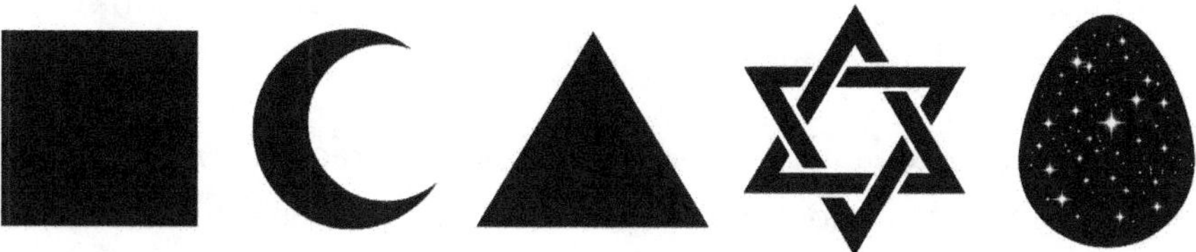

Environment and Duration

Choose a room without noticeable airflow and with a moderate temperature, neither too humid nor too dry. Sit comfortably, open your eyes, and gaze steadily at the chosen symbol without blinking. Begin with about two minutes of *Trāṭaka*, maintaining this duration for several days. Then gradually increase in one-minute increments until you reach five minutes, which should be practiced for about a week, then continue building up to 10 minutes for a week or two, 15 minutes for a month, then 20, 25, and eventually 30 minutes or more. Advanced practitioners can even reach a practice that is several hours long.

You may wonder: *won't my eyes dry out?* No. When the conditions are right, the environment is balanced, and the practice is not forced, the eyes naturally maintain their moisture during the practice.

Relaxed, Not Forced

In the beginning, you may feel the urge to blink, this is completely natural. For the first thirty seconds, it's fine to allow a few blinks. After that, we focus on finding a comfortable way to keep our eyes open without strain.

There are two basic ways to prevent blinking: one is through willpower, which causes tension and burning in the eyes. The other is through *relaxation*, which stills the mind, and it is this option which we should always favor.

Blinking often arises together with thoughts, so rather than fighting the eyes, relax your thoughts. Most thoughts during *Trāṭaka* revolve around discomfort or worry ("Am I hurting my eyes?" "When can I blink?"). As the eyes relax, these thoughts naturally dissolve.

You can relax; no damage is caused by correct practice. *Trāṭaka* can be sustained for long periods. I have practiced this method for over an hour, and some of my colleagues have engaged for up to four hours daily. When both eyes and mind relax, the gaze becomes still, natural, and effortless, and identification with the object deepens so that insights arise on their own.

Finishing the Practice

To close the practice, rub the palms together vigorously until they grow warm and tingly, then gently cup them over your closed eyes without touching the eyeballs, allowing the residual heat to soothe the ocular muscles.

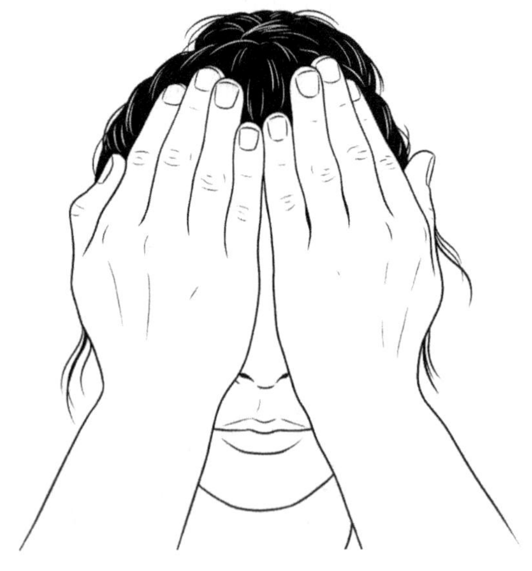

Keep the eyes closed for a few moments. An afterimage of the symbol may appear in complementary colors, if this is the case simply observe it quietly before letting everything relax completely.

Important Notes and Contraindications

1. Remove glasses or contact lenses before practice. Perfect vision is not required—just the ability to clearly distinguish the symbol's shape.
2. As for duration, five minutes is the minimum for noticeable results, fifteen minutes is ideal, and deeper effects tend to appear after thirty minutes or more.
3. Those with glaucoma, elevated intraocular pressure, or retinal or corneal issues must consult an eye doctor before beginning. Describe the practice in detail and get approval, ideally also checking with an experienced yoga teacher familiar with *Trāṭaka*.

Ayurvedic Considerations

According to Ayurveda, one's doṣa (constitution) affects how suitable this technique might be and what precautions are needed,

- **Kapha** types are generally the most stable and usually do not require special precautions.
- **Pitta** types tend to overexert and strain the eyes, to they should progress very slowly, maintain a *soft gaze*, and avoid any irritation or redness.
- **Vāta** types are more sensitive to dryness and should ensure the room is windless and sufficiently humid to prevent itchiness or discomfort.

If your eyes begin to itch, it is a sign that you've overdone the practice. If there is pain, you've gone too far. If you don't know your *doṣa*, consult a questionnaire or an Ayurvedic practitioner before continuing.

Advanced Techniques and Applications

More advanced *Trāṭaka* methods work with the inverted afterimages formed on the retina and rely on specific color arrangements, requiring individualized guidance going beyond the scope of this chapter. Anyone wishing to continue deeper is encouraged to contact an experienced teacher for personal instruction.

Beyond its role in *tattva* recognition, *Trāṭaka* is a powerful tool for enhancing concentration. Even gazing at a simple black dot on a wall can markedly improve focus. I have used *Trāṭaka* to prepare for exams, and it can be a remarkable aid for those with ADHD in cultivating sustained attention.

This concludes our exploration of *Trāṭaka* on the elements—a profound, practical method for developing inner vision and concentration while deepening direct, experiential understanding of the *Tattvas*.

PART IV:
PARALLEL WISDOM TRADITIONS

Chapter 24

Ayurvedic Time Mastery: Aligning with the Rhythms of Nature According to the Ancient Indian Science of Health

I consider that the teaching of Svara Yoga is unique, their emphasis on the biorhythm of alternating nostrils, linked with the alternation between the parasympathetic and sympathetic nervous systems, as well as between the left and the right brain hemispheres is both distinctive to Svara Yoga and scientifically supported as an insight into how the brain functions.

In addition, Svara Yoga's emphasis on how the breath changes based on the flow of the five elements points toward another type of cycle, one that modern science has not fully mapped. Svara Yoga offers concrete techniques to identify where in this cycle we are at any given moment.

But before concluding the teaching of Svara Yoga, I want to turn the focus to some parallel teachings on aligning life with daily rhythms that are drawn from other traditions, both within Hindu tradition and beyond.

To begin, we will start by exploring the Ayurvedic rhythm, or the Ayurvedic clock, closely tied to the science of svara as both are taught within the Hindu tradition.

Understanding Ayurveda: A Brief Overview

Ayurveda is the traditional Indian system of medicine, a vast and intricate field that many readers may already know to some degree. But for those who are new to it, I'll provide a very short introduction — a deliberate oversimplification. If you are well-studied in Ayurveda, please accept my apologies for any inaccuracies that arise from condensing such a rich system into a brief explanation.

Ayurveda, which translates as "the science of life" is an ancient system of holistic healing that originated in India a few thousand years ago. It's one of the oldest and most comprehensive approaches to holistic well-being and rests on several foundational principles.

The Three Doṣas

Ayurveda describes the human constitution in terms of three doṣas: Vāta, Pitta, and Kapha. These doṣas are combinations of the five elements as they manifest in the body and together govern a wide range of physiological and psychological functions.

Vāta is formed from a combination of space and air, Pitta from fire and water, and Kapha from water and earth. According to Ayurveda, every function in the body—and each of the seven bodily tissues that it defines — can be classified as primarily Vāta doṣa, Pitta doṣa, or Kapha doṣa.

Individual Constitution (Prakṛti)

Another fundamental principle in Ayurveda is that each person has an individual constitution called Prakṛti, which we can equate with the interactions between the person's genetic heritage and environmental factors experienced during gestation. This means that each person is born with a unique combination of the doṣas, and this inherent balance shapes physical, mental, and emotional tendencies. Understanding one's Prakṛti is crucial in Ayurveda, as it guides personalized approaches to diet, lifestyle, and treatment choices.

Disease and Imbalance

From the Ayurvedic perspective, disease ultimately arises from an imbalance of the doṣas. Many factors—such as external environments or toxins—can disturb the balance, but illness itself is seen as having too much Vāta, too much Pitta, or too much Kapha. When external bacteria or viruses are involved it is considered that the imbalance creates the opportunity for them to take invade the body and when the imbalance is solved

The Ayurvedic Daily Clock

Most relevant to our discussion, Ayurveda describes a kind of daily clock, similar to the 24-hour circadian rhythm governed by sunrise and sunset, in which the three doṣas take turns predominating. There are times during the day when Vāta doṣa is more dominant, when Pitta is more active, or when Kapha is more pronounced. By aligning Vāta-type actions with Vāta time, Pitta-type actions with Pitta time, and Kapha-type actions with Kapha time, life can come into greater harmony with this natural rhythm.

The Three Doṣas in Detail

Let's now briefly describe the three doṣas, and then introduce the Ayurvedic clock, so we can better understand how Ayurveda recommends aligning our actions with the various hours of the day.

Vāta Doṣa

Vāta is composed, as I mentioned, of the space and air elements, which makes it light, dry, and cold. People with a predominant Vāta constitution often have a lean physique, dry skin, and often experience cold hands and feet.

Emotionally, Vāta individuals tend to be creative, imaginative, and quick-thinking, yet when imbalanced they are prone to anxiety, restlessness, and indecision.

Vāta governs movement in the body, including: breathing, muscle contractions, and circulation, and it supports mental agility, creativity, and sensory perception. It is primarily located in the colon (gas), the bones (due to their porous nature), the lungs, and especially the nervous system, where the nerves carry the mental vibration of Vāta.

When Vāta is out of balance, it can manifest as anxiety disorders, insomnia, constipation, arthritis, joint pain, various nerve disorders, and dry skin conditions.

Pitta Doṣa

Pitta is made of the fire and water elements and is characterized as hot and sharp. In terms of body humours, it corresponds to bile. As hot, transformative "water", Pitta underlies the body's capacity for change and chemical reaction.

Pitta is associated with the digestive and endocrine system—all the hormones and digestive juices, metabolism, and the processes of transformation. It regulates body temperature and appetite while driving the production of various enzymes in the body.

Individuals with dominant Pitta usually have a moderate build and warm skin and may be prone to conditions related to excessive heat. Psychologically, Pitta individuals are intelligent, ambitious, and goal-oriented, but when imbalanced can become irritable, critical, and overly competitive.

Pitta is normally located in the small intestines, stomach, liver, spleen, blood, and eyes. When Pitta goes out of balance, it can lead to acid reflux, ulcers, inflammation, eczema, liver disorders, hypertension, and excessive sweating.

Kapha Doṣa

Finally, Kapha is composed of the earth and water elements, and is characterized as heavy, stable, and cool. It governs stability, structure, and lubrication in the body, regulating growth, strength, and the immune system. In the classical theory of humours, Kapha corresponds to phlegm or mucus.

Kapha-dominant individuals tend to have a sturdy build, soft skin, and a tendency to retain moisture. Kapha is located mainly in the chest, throat, head, lymph, and fat tissues, and when it becomes imbalanced it can give rise to respiratory conditions, obesity, diabetes, sinusitis, sluggish digestion, and excessive mucus production.

Summary of the Three Doṣas

Doṣa	Elements	Qualities	Physical Traits	Mental/ Emotional Traits	Primary Locations	Imbalance Conditions
Vāta	Space + Air	Light dry cold	Lean physique, dry skin, cold extremities	Creative, quick thinking, imaginative; prone to anxiety and restlessness	Colon, bones, lungs, nervous system	Anxiety, insomnia, constipation, arthritis, nerve disorders
Pitta	Fire + Water	Hot sharp	Moderate build, warm skin	Intelligent, ambitious, goal-oriented; can become irritable and critical	Small intestines, stomach, liver, spleen, blood, eyes	Acid reflux, ulcers, inflammation, eczema, hypertension
Kapha	Earth + Water	Heavy stable cool	Sturdy build, soft skin	Calm, nurturing; can become lethargic and stubborn	Chest, throat, head, lymph, fat tissues	Respiratory issues, obesity, diabetes, sinusitis, sluggish digestion

Living According to Your Doṣa

Ayurveda offers practical guidelines for living in harmony with your doṣa. If your constitution is Vāta, typical advice includes going to sleep early and avoiding behaviors or foods that increase wind in the body—such as gas-producing foods, eating while standing, and tendencies toward excessive worrying. If you are more prone to Pitta imbalance, you would be advised to avoid spicy foods, limit strong sun exposure, and in general steer clear of things that further inflame Pitta. And if your constitution is Kapha, recommendations often include not oversleeping and reducing sweets and dairy products, which increase heaviness and mucus.

For anyone practicing yoga, checking your Ayurvedic constitution is especially valuable. Once you know it, you can consciously work to align diet and lifestyle with your physical makeup, which tends to create more comfort in the body and greater ease in daily life.

The Ayurvedic Clock: Aligning with Daily Rhythms

Ayurveda also describes a biological clock, determined by the sun's position in the sky. Beginning at 6 A.M. it divides the day into six four-hour segments each characterized by a predominant doṣa. Thus over the course of each day, our body cycles twice through phases dominated by Vāta, Kapha, and Pitta. When our daily routines are aligned with these cycles, well-being, happiness, and health are supported, while consistent deviation can disrupt our health and contribute to disease.

Starting From 6 A.M. to 10 A.M., Kapha predominates. From 10 A.M. to 2 P.M., as the sun rises higher and heat increases, Pitta governs. From 2 P.M. to 6 P.M., the atmosphere shifts into a calmer Vāta period leading toward sunset. From 6 P.M. to 10 P.M., Kapha becomes dominant again. From 10 P.M. to 2 A.M., Pitta rules once more and from 2 A.M. to 6 A.M., the final Vāta phase completes the cycle before sunrise.

Time Period	Dominant Doṣa	Primary Organ/System	Key Activities Recommended
2 A.M. - 6 A.M.	Vāta	Colon, bladder	Wake up (ideally 4 A.M.), evacuate, bathe, meditate, spiritual practice
6 A.M. - 10 A.M.	Kapha	Lungs, pancreas	Exercise, movement, light breakfast (around 8 A.M.)
10 A.M. - 2 P.M.	Pitta	Small intestines, stomach, heart	Work, main meal (at noon), digest
2 P.M. - 6 P.M.	Vāta	Liver, gallbladder	Creative work, light dinner (before 6 P.M.)
6 P.M. - 10 P.M.	Kapha	Lungs, pancreas	Wind down, light exercise, evening routine, sleep by 10 P.M.
10 P.M. - 2 A.M.	Pitta	Small intestines, stomach, heart	Sleep, body repair, dream processingv

Detailed Journey Through the Ayurvedic Day

Let's now look at what Ayurveda recommends for each of these time frames, beginning at 2 A.M. and ending at 6 A.M., The period during which it is recommended to wake up.

2 - 6 A.M.: Night Vāta Time

Ayurveda begins its practical day at 2 A.M., when the night Vāta period starts and the body's prāṇa moves to the spleen. This shift can potentially stir emotions such as anger, though it is generally still sleep time.

Around 4 A.M., prāṇa moves to the colon and bladder, making this the best time to wake, evacuate the bladder and bowels, bathe, and groom in anticipation of the day. Ayurveda believes that if we become imbalanced in this moment, we will generate anxiety.

This early Vāta window is particularly supportive for exploring our spiritual connection with the universe. Ayurveda therefore places strong emphasis on using morning rituals for introspection, cleansing routines, meditation, āsana practice, prayer, and other spiritual activities.

6 - 10 A.M.: Morning Kapha Time

At 6 A.M. the cycle enters Kapha time. From 6 to 8 A.M., the prāṇa moves into the lungs, a phase in which imbalance can manifest as grief and sadness, and because Kapha is heavy, Ayurveda recommends against waking up after 6 A.M. Doing so often leaves one feeling more sluggish, tired, and inclined to stay in bed.

To counter Kapha's inertia, this period is recommended for movement: exercise, going outside, and actively starting our day. Around 8 A.M., prāṇa moves into the pancreas, making it an excellent time to eat your breakfast—ideally a light one, especially for Kapha constitutions, as digestion is slower during Kapha and heavy food can weigh the system down. Kapha is also quite social, so this is a good time to connect with others and build relationships.

10 - 2 P.M.: Midday Pitta Time

At 10 A.M., we enter Pitta time, as prāṇa flows into the small intestines and stomach. If imbalanced, this phase can breed anxiety and anger. This is a very good time for digestion, and because Pitta governs transformation, it is also the prime time for acting, both internally and externally, to create change, making it an ideal period for focused work and getting tasks done.

Around midday, prāṇa moves into the heart, activating both joy and deep-rooted, unresolved emotions. Ayurveda considers noon the best time to have the main meal of the day, followed by two hours for digestion, as this is when the body can most effectively handle heavier foods that provide sustained nourishment.

At the same time, make sure to take a conscious break during and remember that excessive Pitta may increase interpersonal tensions. This makes it wise to protect a bit of space for yourself during this time if needed.

2 - 6 P.M.: Afternoon Vāta Time

At 2 P.M., the afternoon Vāta time begins, with prāṇa entering the liver and gallbladder and, when out of balance, potentially triggering anger, hatred, and resentment. This remains a good time for digestion, but the quality of Vāta also strongly colors mental activity.

As Vāta governs movement, the nervous system, and sensory experience, a rested and balanced body-mind can use this time to be creative and to think abstractly about life's problems. If rest is lacking, however, this phase often brings fatigue, energy dips, sugar cravings, spaciness, or being easily distracted.

To make the most of it, Ayurveda suggests creating a calm atmosphere and reducing stimulation: taking a walk, drinking tea, or practicing relaxation, and when stable, harnessing this time of creativity to your advantage for brainstorming, starting new projects, reading, and meaningful connections with people. However, avoid trying to cram all remaining tasks into this slot, because that would aggravate Vāta and fuel excess worry.

Ayurveda further recommends having dinner at the end of this period, a little before 6 P.M., and keeping it light. Eating dinner around 5 P.M. may feel early by modern standards, yet it supports easier digestion and better balance going into the evening.

6 - 10 P.M.: Evening Kapha Time

At 6 P.M., the second Kapha period of the day begins with prāṇa moving into the lungs which may generate grief or sadness if imbalanced. This is the best time to wind down, meet family and friends, connect with loved ones, and enjoy the simple comforts that Kapha brings.

This window also supports grounding exercise—not intense, but practices that stretch and relax the body, such as yoga, walking, or swimming. If you did not eat around 5 P.M., you can take a very light dinner early in this Kapha time.

It's best to minimize stimulation from screens, phones, and computers so the system can gradually move towards sleep. While Pitta time suits spontaneity and Vāta time requiring gentle structure, this evening Kapha period benefits from one single, steady, simple routine.

Around 8 P.M., prāṇa shifts into the pancreas and, when disturbed, can increase attachment, which is another reason to lean into a clear evening routine that culminates in going to bed by 10 P.M. Ayurveda explicitly recommends never going to sleep later than this time.

10 - 2 A.M.: Night Pitta Time

At 10 P.M., the prāṇa again enters the small intestines and stomach, marking the beginning of the second Pitta period, a time when imbalances can breed anger and anxiety. Because Pitta is fiery and activating, staying awake past 10 P.M. often triggers a "second wind", a kind of rush of energy that may keep you up much later than is healthy. And so, we are invited to remain asleep throughout this entire second Pitta window.

From midnight to 2 A.M., prāṇa moves into the heart. This phase supports experiencing the joys of dreaming and metabolizing unresolved emotional material in anticipation of waking up refreshed, somewhere between 4 and 6 A.M. the next morning.

Adapting the Ayurvedic Clock to Your Life

The Ayurvedic clock offers a wonderful way to align with a solar-based biorhythm, yet it must also be adapted intelligently to where and how you live.

You might wonder how this clock relates to places across the world where the sun rises very early or sets very late. The truth is that human beings maintain an inherent 24-hour circadian rhythm regardless of their location in the world, a pattern biologically baked over millions of years when humanity largely lived around the equator. So even in far northern or southern latitudes, where daylight shifts dramatically, this inner 24-hour rhythm remains the baseline.

However, in regions with very early sunrises or very late sunsets, the varying length of daylight can skew strict application of the Ayurvedic schedule, but the fundamental 24-hour rhythm still applies. For this reason, the emphasis is less on copying exact clock times and more on attuning to phases of the day—light, heat, and quiet—that approximate the Kapha, Pitta, and Vāta periods in your own environment.

A practical way to incorporate this into your practice is to implement things slowly, making one change at a time rather than overhauling your entire routine. For example, you can start by waking up a little bit earlier, aiming to rise before 6 A.M., and dedicating that pre-6 A.M. window to Vāta-supportive activities such as cleansing, meditation, and gentle practice, then slowly experiment with adjusting meals and see how each shift feels to your body and mind. Over time, this gentle experimentation reveals the timings that truly work for you, turning the Ayurvedic clock from a rigid schedule into a living, responsive guide.

Chapter 25
Qi Flow Mastery: Harnessing Vital Energy through the Chinese Clock

Introduction to the Chinese Body Clock

Now that we have explored the Ayurvedic clock, in this chapter I want to describe a closely related model from another tradition that enriches the study of Svara: traditional Chinese medicine. This system works with yin and yang, which correspond conceptually to the left and right Svaras, or more precisely, to the principles of the Iḍā nāḍī and the Piṅgalā nāḍī. Even though traditional Chinese medicine does not describe breath moving through the left and right nostrils as such.

Just as Ayurveda describes a 24-hour body clock in which prāṇa moves from organ to organ, Chinese medical treatises describe a parallel clock in which their equivalent of prāṇa—termed qi—circulates through different organs in sequence. As prāṇa, or qi, concentrates in each organ in turn, different actions become more or less beneficial. Based on this understanding, the tradition recommends which actions to undertake or avoid at particular times.

Choosing Between the Ayurvedic and Chinese Clocks

When the Ayurvedic and Chinese clocks are compared, we will see that they align on many accounts but also differ on some details, which naturally raises the question: which clock should you follow? My recommendation is simple.

If your main practices and techniques arise from the Chinese framework, such as qigong, tai chi, kung fu, and other such practices, you are already tuning your body to the rhythms described by this tradition. Working with qi in ways taught by these methods naturally aligns you with the Chinese organ click, so in that case, I would recommend that you use the Chinese qi body clock as your primary reference.

If, on the other hand, your core practices come from the Indian tradition, such as yoga and its associated meditations, then your body cycles are already being harmonized with the patterns described in the Indian, and specifically Ayurvedic, tradition. In that situation, then I would recommend using the Ayurvedic clock as your main guide.

The Twenty-Four-Hour Qi Cycle

Let's review the Chinese qi clock starting at roughly the same point as the Ayurvedic clock, around 3 A.M.

3-5 A.M.: The Lungs (Yin Metal)

From 3 to 5 A.M., the qi is said to reside in the lungs, and their energy is at a peak. This is ideally a time to remain asleep, supported by soft, deep, rhythmic breathing that helps process emotions such as grief that is often associated with the lungs.

This phase is considered a time of embodiment and inspiration, connected with yin or lunar qi and the metal element. While this often parallels the Indian element of ākāśa, or ether, because the Chinese element system developed somewhat independently, equivalences are sometimes hard to make. In some cases, one Chinese element may fit its equivalent perfectly—like fire and fire—but others will see discrepancies. Metal often corresponds to the element of ether, though can also resemble water or air.

Signs like shortness of breath, lung disorders, colds and flu, allergies, asthma, dry skin, depression, or excessive crying may indicate deficiency or imbalance of lung qi, making this time of day particularly important to honor and observe.

5-7 A.M.: The Large Intestine (Yang Metal)

From 5 to 7 A.M., the body's qi moves to the large intestines, whose activity becomes most prominent. The body is naturally prepared to wake and start a new day, and, in a healthy state, empty its bowels soon after rising, clearing waste accumulated overnight to create a fresh internal start.

This period is framed as a time of transformation and consciously embracing a new day, still connected to the metal element but now with yang predominating. If we conceptually compared this with the Indian system, the yang metal phase would loosely correspond to a preference for breathing through the right nostril, even though such nostril-specific language is not mentioned in the Chinese tradition itself.

The large intestines are said to be especially sensitive to anxiety, so this is an important time to avoid cultivating anxious thoughts and to support a calm, unhurried start to the day.

7-9 A.M.: The Stomach (Yang Earth)

Between 7 and 9 A.M., the qi moves into the stomach, creating a sense of balance and signaling a natural time for arrival and grounding. In traditional Chinese medicine, this is considered the optimal window to have breakfast, specifically a big breakfast, because digestion and absorption are at their peak when the stomach holds the greatest concentration of qi.

At this time, the dominant element shifts from metal to earth in its yang aspect, continuing the yang energy from the large intestines, but now transitioning from yang metal to yang earth.

9-11 A.M.: The Spleen (Yin Earth)

From 9 to11 A.M., the qi moves to the spleen, which still belongs to the earth element but now in yin mode rather than yang. The spleen is understood to convert the food we eat into "food for thought", making this an excellent time for focused work and physical exercise.

The spleen is also connected with worrying and overthinking, so excessive mental work, dwelling, or fixation on a singular issue may cause spleen-related imbalance. Symptoms such as fatigue, loss of appetite, mucus discharge, poor digestion, abdominal distension, loose stools or diarrhea, weak muscles, pale lips, easy bruising, excess menstrual bleeding, or other bleeding tendencies may all indicate spleen qi disharmony, suggesting that extra care with this point of the day should receive your attention.

11 A.M.-1 P.M.: The Heart (Yin Fire)

Between 11 A.M. and 1 P.M., at high noon, the qi concentrates in the heart, the yin organ of the fire element. This is also when the day reaches its peak Yang expression (with midnight being the peak Yin time). During this window, the body emphasizes circulating nutrients absorbed from food throughout the entire system, and the heart's association with joy and soulful purpose is highlighted.

However, when heart fire is overstimulated, it can lead to agitation, insomnia, and palpitations, while deficiency or imbalance may show up as lack of enthusiasm, low vitality, mental restlessness, depression, insomnia and despair, excessive dreaming, or poor long-term memory.

1-3 P.M.: The Small Intestine (Yang Fire)

From 1 to 3 P.M., the qi transitions to the small intestines, the yang aspect of the fire element. This organ is responsible for "separating the clear from the turbid"—physically, it filters nutrients toward the kidneys or waste toward the large intestine; mentally, it helps us distinguish between what is useful and what is fluff.

In traditional Chinese medicine, this is considered the appropriate time to have lunch or finish digesting a midday meal, as the fire energy helps "cook" and transform food into energy. Because of its role in discernment, this is a phase where the gentle slowing of the day can bring clarity of thought. If you feel a "brain fog" or indecisiveness during this window, it may indicate a deficiency in the small intestine's ability to sort through the day's information and nutrition.

3-5 P.M.: The Bladder (Yang Water)

Between 3 and 5 P.M., the qi shifts into the bladder, expressing the water element in its yang form. As the longest meridian in the body, running from the eyes, over the head, and down the entire back, the bladder is framed as a massive reservoir of support for the other organs.

This period is well-suited to routine tasks or "wrapping up" work, but it is also a common time for a "3 P.M. slump" if one is dehydrated or if kidney/bladder qi is low. It is an essential time to hydrate adequately to support the filtration of fluids. Because the bladder meridian governs the nervous system's response along the spine, a lack of energy now may manifest as back pain or a desire for salt. Traditional practitioners often suggest this as a peak time for learning or memory-based tasks, provided the body is properly fueled and watered.

5-7 P.M.: The Kidneys (Yin Water)

From 5 to7 P.M., the qi flows to the kidneys, which are the yin water organs considered the root of all energy in the Chinese organ system. This is an excellent time to eat a light, nourishing evening meal and for gently switching off, to socialize, to laugh, and to unwind.

The kidneys are described as key organs central to reproduction, growth, development, and maturation, working with the lungs in water metabolism and respiration and closely connected to bones, teeth, ears, and head hair.

Emotionally, they are especially vulnerable to fear and are linked with weak willpower, insecurity, aloofness, and isolation. Extreme fright can impair their ability to hold qi, potentially leading to various conditions such as frequent urination, incontinence, night sweats, dry mouth, poor short-term memory, lower back pain, ringing in the ears (tinnitus), hearing loss, other ear conditions, premature gray hair, hair loss, and osteoporosis.

7-9 P.M.: The Pericardium (Yin Ministerial Fire)

From 7 to 9 P.M., the qi moves into the ministerial fire in its yin aspect, residing in the pericardium. Often called the "Heart Protector" or the "King's Bodyguard", its role is to shield the heart, considered the emperor of the body, from excessive emotional shocks, trauma, and the daily grind of life. This is an especially supportive time for activities that nourish the heart such as: socializing with loved ones, creating art or music, dancing, or sharing a relaxed dinner.

Because the pericardium governs emotional intimacy and healthy boundaries, it is the ideal time to "close the gates" to the stresses of the outside world and focus on connection. If the pericardium is out of balance, you may experience difficulty expressing emotions, feelings of extreme vulnerability, or, on the other hand a sense of emotional numbness and detachment. Physically, disharmony during these hours often manifests as chest tightness, palpitations, or a restless energy that makes it difficult to wind down. By engaging in light, joyful activities now, you help calm your nervous system and prepare the spirit for the deep rest of the upcoming night.

9-11 P.M.: The Triple Burner/Sanjiao (Yang Ministerial Fire)

From 9 and 11 P.M., the qi shifts into its yang ministerial fire expression within the triple burner, or sanjiao, a functional, energetic system that relates to the regulation and distribution of metabolic and physiological processes in the body rather than a single anatomical organ.

The triple burner has three parts: upper (respiration and chest organ communication), middle (digestion and transformation of foods and fluids in the abdominal region), and lower (pelvic functions like reproduction, urination, and elimination). Together they regulate metabolism, fluid movement, and heat, while also supporting mental clarity, emotional stability, and mind–body harmony. This interval is an ideal time to wind down and let the system quiet. Gentle stretching, meditation, reading, or cuddling are recommended, coinciding with the beginning of melatonin secretion in the circadian rhythm that prepares us for sleep.

11 P.M.-1 A.M.: The Gallbladder (Yang Wood)

Here is the refined and expanded section for the Gallbladder. I have kept it concise while adding the physical indicators and the "Wood" element context to match your other entries.

11 P.M.-1 A.M.: The Gallbladder (Yang Wood)

From 11 P.M. to 1 A.M., qi moves into the gallbladder, representing the yang aspect of the wood element. This phase parallels the air element in Indian and Greek traditions and is regarded as a time for deep unconscious processing and cellular regeneration. Physically, this is when the body focuses on building blood and excreting bile to process fats.

The gallbladder is known as the "Official of Decision Making". In a balanced state, it provides the courage and judgment needed to take action; however, an imbalance often manifests as chronic indecisiveness, low self-esteem, or lingering resentment. Because this window is essential for the "resetting" of the nervous system, it reinforces the guidance that this is a period during which we should be in deep sleep. Waking or restlessness during these hours may indicate unresolved frustration or a struggle to find a clear direction in life.

1-3 A.M.: The Liver (Yin Wood)

From 1-3 A.M., the qi cycle closes as energy moves into the liver, expressing the yin aspect of the wood element. This is considered the best time for deep sleep and dreaming—a window of time for profound recovery and, in many traditions, for receiving deeper spiritual guidance.

The liver is closely connected to anger, and strong angry emotions can cause liver energy to surge upward, resulting in headaches, dizziness, or high blood pressure. In traditional Chinese medicine, the liver governs the smooth flow of qi and blood throughout the body, regulates bile secretions, stores blood, and connects with the tendons, nails, and eyes.

When liver qi becomes disturbed by emotions such as anger, resentment, frustration, irritability, or bitterness, it can manifest as breast distension, menstrual pain, headaches, irritability, outbursts of anger, dizziness, dry or red eyes and other eye conditions, as well as tendinitis. Frequently waking during this 1–3 A.M. interval is interpreted as a sign of having too much yang energy or underlying liver imbalance, indicating that this area of health deserves some attention.

Time	Organ	Element	Yin/ Yang	Key Functions	Associated Emotions
3-5 A.M.	Lungs	Metal	Yin	Respiration, immunity	Grief, Sadness
5-7 A.M.	Large Intestine	Metal	Yang	Elimination, "letting go"	Guilt, Stuckness
7-9 A.M.	Stomach	Earth	Yang	Digestion, receiving	Worry, Despair
9-11 A.M.	Spleen	Earth	Yin	Transformation of Qi	Worry, Pensiveness
11 A.M.-1 P.M.	Heart	Fire	Yin	Blood & spirit (Shen)	Joy, Enthusiasm
1-3 P.M.	Small Intestine	Fire	Yang	Sorting clear/turbid	Insecurity, Vulnerability
3-5 P.M.	Bladder	Water	Yang	Liquid waste, storage	Fear, Irritation
5-7 P.M.	Kidneys	Water	Yin	Essence (Jing), filter	Fear, Insecurity
7-9 P.M.	Pericardium	Ministerial Fire	Yin	Heart protection	Compassion, Intimacy
9-11 P.M.	Triple Burner	Ministerial Fire	Yang	Metabolism, Thermoregulation	Overwhelm, Hopelessness
11 P.M.-1 A.M.	Gallbladder	Wood	Yang	Decisions, bile	Indecision, Bitterness
1-3 A.M.	Liver	Wood	Yin	Detox, smooth flow	Anger, Frustration

PART V: SPECIALIZED APPLICATIONS

Chapter 25
Sacred Beginnings: Svara Wisdom for Pregnancy and Childbirth

In these final chapters, I want to address the more divinatory aspects of the *Śiva Svarodaya*, as well as some subjects that might be controversial. I mention them for your general knowledge. In this chapter, I'm going to discuss the family planning aspect of the *Śiva Svarodaya.*

I have placed this chapter towards the end not because this is an unimportant topic, but because I feel that the *Śiva Svarodaya* is not entirely accurate; I feel that it presents a very patriarchal view of the universe and find that I don't overly trust this portion of its teachings. The Svarodaya Śāstra, in my belief, was written mainly by men for men. This is the language that the text assumes. And since it's only females who give birth in the human race, I believe that any kind of teaching that talks about this function should be written and guided by those who can actually do it. And that was unlikely to have happened here.

As such, I don't really like this part of the text, but I will share it with you, and you can decide for yourselves. And of course, if this is triggering for you, or if you don't want to hear what very ancient (probably male) authors had to say about this subject, then please skip ahead.

I will note that of all the traditions in India, the tantric tradition out of which the Svarodaya Śāstra was born was indeed accepting of women as teachers, as masters, and as lineage holders. But my feeling from the text is that it is nevertheless male-centric and patrilineal, and so, as I said, I don't feel trust in this part of the teaching.

Ancient Theories of Conception

As I mentioned, the work presents a very archaic view of pregnancy. The Svarodaya Śāstra's belief is that pregnancy is caused by the meeting of the menstrual blood with the semen in the uterus, and that somehow the semen causes the menstrual blood to congeal and turn into the fetus.

The Svarodaya Śāstra goes on to instruct on multiple ways to determine the sex of the child. But before teaching these techniques, it posits that the ultimate cause for birthing a male is when the semen is larger in quantity than the menstrual blood, and that the cause for birthing a female is when the menstrual blood is greater in quantity than the semen.

The Svarodaya Śāstra believes that conception is possible for sixteen nights after the menses, and another determining factor is whether the copulation was performed on an even or odd night after menses. According to it, if conception takes place on an even night after menses, then a female will be created, and if conception takes place on an odd night after menses, then a male will be created.

Conception, as we now know, can happen a few days after the joining of the female and the male. But according to the *Śiva Svarodaya* and the *Svara cintāmaṇi*, conception is supposed to happen at the moment of copulation.

The Sixteen Nights: Traditional Predictions

The *Svara cintāmaṇi* shares the following predictions based on the night of conception after menstruation:

Night	Sex	Predicted Characteristics
4th	Male	Short-lived and poverty-stricken
5th	Female	Will have many children
6th	Male	Will have medium effects
7th	Female	Will be unchaste
8th	Male	Will be wealthy
9th	Female	Will be chaste
10th	Male	Will be a lord
11th	Female	Will be irreligious
12th	Male	Will be good
13th	Female	Will associate with persons of other castes
14th	Male	Will be grateful, charitable, interested in yoga philosophy, an observer of strict fasts and a jewel of the world because of his superior qualities
15th	Female	Will be extremely lucky, will be having many children, will be chaste and will be born in a royal family or wedded to a government servant
16th	Male	Will be a truthful controller of senses, learned and equal to all beings

As you can see, the text is quite misogynistic and male-oriented, but this is indeed the information that it provides.

Modern Scientific Perspectives

Maybe there is some truth to the idea that females and males are conceived differently depending on the day of conception. Of course, with modern statistics we could actually test this. As far as I know, no one has.

There have been various scholarly studies examining the day of conception in relation to ovulation, and their results are conflicting. Some research shows that when conception happens on the day of ovulation it leads to more male children, and some research shows the absolute opposite. So, the main conclusion at present is that we just don't know. Maybe the sex of the child changes based on the day of conception, and maybe not.

The research found has not focused on even or odd days, as the *Svara cintāmaṇi* teaches, but rather on the timing of the joining of male and female in relation to ovulation, whether it is before or after ovulation—though the timing addressed in research could, theoretically, align with days out as *Svara cintāmaṇi* addresses.

Most of the knowledge circulating today suggests that to conceive a girl, the joining should happen between the end of menstruation and three days before ovulation, while abstaining for two to three days before ovulation. In order to conceive a boy, the joining is said to be best on the day of ovulation and during the following three days. This timing is said to be related to the ability of individual spermatozoon to swim: those carrying the Y chromosome are considered better short-term swimmers, while those carrying the X chromosome are considered better long-term swimmers and can survive longer. But, as mentioned, the research here is mixed.

Svara-Based Methods for Sex Determination

Another teaching within the *Śiva Svarodaya* indicates that to determine the sex of a child, one should look at the svaras as they flow in both the female and the male being joined. A woman wanting a male child should initiate joining during her fertile period when her left nostril is active and her partner's right nostril is active. It is also suggested that the joining take place when the earth element is active.

For the conception of a girl, the woman's right nostril should be flowing and the partner's left nostril should be active, and should occur during the activation of the water element. The Svara Śāstra also teaches that if getting pregnant is difficult, it is recommended for the female to join with the male either when her central channel has just opened or when her prāṇa is flowing in the fire element of the solar svara.

Elemental Influences on Pregnancy

Trigger warning: The following section contains information about pregnancy in general and about unsuccessful pregnancies. If you might be uncomfortable reading this, you can skip ahead. Again, this is not information that feels very trustworthy for me personally. It certainly has not been tested, and these are ideas that could be examined much more easily with modern science. But this is what is the text we are studying presents.

I invite you to consider the bits which interest you and to put the rest aside. You can keep the information here simply for your general knowledge. Hopefully you find these teachings at least interesting, if not insightful, and that you enjoy engaging with it. I include this section because I believe that some people may find it meaningful, and leaving it out would feel like leaving the book incomplete.

The teachings the Svara Śāstra presents on how the different elements affect pregnancy are described in two slightly different versions within the texts:

Version One: Elemental Effects

Element	Effect on Offspring
Air	The offspring, being a son, will be morose
Water	He will be famous in all directions and will have a pleasurable life
Fire	There will be either an abortion or the baby will be short-lived
Earth	He will enjoy material life and be handsome and wealthy

Version Two: Expanded Elemental Effects

Element	Sex	Effect
Water	Son	Will be wealthy, happy, and an enjoyer of material life, and his wealth will ever remain with him
Ether	—	There will be an abortion
Earth	Son	A beautiful son will be born
Water	Daughter	A daughter will be born
Other elements	—	There will be either an abortion or the child will die soon after birth

Chapter 26
The Final Transition: Tantric Wisdom on Predicting the Moment of Passing

Introduction: Humanity's Ancient Preoccupation with Death

In this chapter, I want to address a subject that has always preoccupied human beings, and is covered in many of the Svarodaya texts: the prediction of the time of death.

The fear of death is one of the oldest and deepest human fears, and the uncertainty of what follows the moment of death has been the cause of anxieties for centuries. Even for those who believe in a spiritual afterlife or in reincarnation, knowing the moment of death is considered vital because it gives a person the opportunity to prepare themselves for this transition. Thus, many traditional tantric texts teach various methodologies for determining the time of one's passing.

Historical Sources and Context

The information on this subject found in the *Śiva Svarodaya* is in my view not original. In my research, I have uncovered earlier mentions that probably serve as the basis for some of the teachings found within the work. Many techniques taught in the *Śiva Svarodaya* around predicting one's death also appear in more elaborated forms in works such as the *Bardo Thödol* (the Tibetan Book of the Dead), the *Kālacakra Tantra*, which is an 11th-century Buddhist Tantra, the 7th-century Svacchanda Tantra, and the Kalottara Tantra.

When attempting to determine which text is the source and which text copied ideas from where, we look at the richness and complexity of the information. When comparing, for example, the *Śiva Svarodaya* with the *Bardo Thödol*, there are certain techniques for which the *Śiva Svarodaya* gives only one example, while the Tibetan Book of the Dead provides five or ten examples. The information is therefore more robust and complete in the Tibetan Book of the Dead, which suggests that it was the origin source and that the *Śiva Svarodaya* replicated just part of the original material.

Why mention this? The material here will be presented mostly as it appears in the *Śiva Svarodaya*. If this subject interests you, I invite you to pick up a copy of the Tibetan Book of the Dead: First Complete Translation, where you will find much more detailed information. In the following sections, however, the main categories of predictive techniques for death will be outlined, along with what the *Śiva Svarodaya* has to say on this subject.

Observing the Flow of Svara

Basic Principles of Continuous Flow

First and foremost, the *Śiva Svarodaya* tells us to observe the flow of the svaras when exploring these predictive questions. It says that if the flow of svara is continuous, night and day, through one nostril, death will happen in three years; in other words, if the svara doesn't change for 24 hours and stays on the same nostril, death is likely to occur within three years.

If the solar svara of a person flows continuously for two consecutive days and nights—specifically the solar, right nostril svara–it is said that the person has only two years of life remaining. When the same nāḍī flows continuously for up to three nights, one year of life is left. It's not entirely clear here whether "same nāḍī" means simply either left or right, or "the same nāḍī" as in the previous verse, i.e., the right nostril.

The Kalottara Tantra adds:

> "If only one nāḍī flows after midnight, life is endangered, but if it lasts only two yāmas (6 hours), the person survive"
>
> (Kalottara-1300, 8.142)

Alternating Day and Night Patterns

The next verse continues by saying that when the lunar svara of a person flows continuously at night, and the solar svara flows continuously during the day, death will occur within six months. So if the left nostril flows for 12 hours at night and the right nostril for 12 hours during day, then death is said to come within six months.

Extended Duration Predictions

Elsewhere in the text, it states that if the solar svara flows continuously for 16 days, death will come by the last of the even numbered days of that month. If the solar svara flows at full strength constantly and the lunar svara does not flow at all, death will occur within 15 days. On the other hand, if the lunar svara flows at full strength constantly and the solar svara does not flow at all, death will occur within one month.

Tibetan and Kālacakra Elaborations

The Tibetan Book of the Dead offers a different way of looking at these prediction, involving checking the breath around the vernal equinox, where it's supposed to flow for three days through one nostril and then three days through the other. This method is quite complex, so I will not detail it here. If you want a more elaborate explanation, the *Kālacakra*

Tantra, in its second chapter, contains extensive information about the signs of death and how they appear.

The whole scheme presented in the Tibetan Book of the Dead is outlined in the table below, connecting breathing through the nostrils and the time of death:

Duration of Left Nostril Flow	**Time Until Death**
1 day	36 months (3 years)
3 days	30 months
6 days	27 months
9 days	24 months
12 days	21 months
15 days	18 months
18 days	15 months
21 days	12 months
24 days	9 months
27 days	6 months
30 days	3 months
33 days	End of 3 months

General Physical Signs of Approaching Death

The *Śiva Svarodaya*, as well as the Tibetan Book of the Dead, the *Kālacakra Tantra*, and other tantras, speak about various additional signs of impending death. For example, if the middle three fingers do not bend, if the throat becomes dry without illness, and if there appears to be loss of memory shown by asking the same questions again and again, then death is said to come within six months.

Another example is that if one feels pain in the palm or at the root of the tongue, or if the blood becomes blackish, or if one does not look toward the place where one is pricked, then one will only live up to seven months.

Observational Science of Aging

These types of predictions are very general and also correlate to how people age and how responsiveness to the environment decreases over time. If we went into elder-care homes today, we would certainly see people coming to very similar conclusions.

Some of the information here—about loss of joint flexibility, diminishing eyesight, the inability to see the bridge of the nose or the eyebrows, and the cooling of the extremities—are all signs that people working in such homes would likely recognize. From practical experience, I can tell you that most of these do seem to apply, in a broad way, to people who are reaching the end of their lives.

There's not much mysticism here. It's largely a collection of observations. You could call it a kind of observational science, carried out in an unsystematic way, about a thousand years ago or so.

The Eye-Pressing Technique

Beyond these general signs, there are two particularly interesting techniques in the *Śiva Svarodaya* that are probably taken directly from the Tibetan. To describe them clearly, I'm going to rely on the Tibetan presentation because it seems that some errors may have crept into the *Śiva Svarodaya* as it was compiled.

Basic Method from *Śiva Svarodaya*

The first of these techniques is a method in which you close your eyes and gently press on them with the fingers. The *Śiva Svarodaya* summarizes this in a single verse: "If after pressing the corners of the eyes slightly with the fingers and gazing steadfastly at a blank space, one does not see any spot of light, one will die within 10 days".

I invite you to explore this yourself: close your eyes and then direct your gaze in a particular direction. For example, if you are going to touch the right eye, look toward the right. Then, from the side of the nose, place your finger on the left side of the right eyelid, pressing gently on the left side of the eyeball so that it is pushed slightly to the right. You will then see a little spot of light.

If you simply press the eye and look at a blank space, you will notice a kind of dot or circle of light that lingers in your visual field. This is purely physiological. The text basically says that if you don't see this, it means the eye is losing a certain suppleness, and that this loss happens only shortly before death. In such a case, death is said to occur within ten days.

Elaborated Tibetan Method

In the Tibetan Book of the Dead, the same idea appears in a much more elaborate form. There it states: "If the circles of light which appear are absent from the lower part of the left eye, this indicates that one may die after six months. But if they are absent from the upper part of the left eye, that means death will happen in three months. If the same circles are absent from the direction of the left nostril, this indicates that one may die after one month. If they are absent from the direction of the left ear, that means that one may die after two months".

Here the instruction is to work with the left eye. There are two possible ways to interpret how to do this. The first is simply to press on the eye and then look at a blank surface, observing whether circles of light appear in the different "corners" of the visual field. If a circle is missing in any one of these areas, death is said to occur within a corresponding time.

In this interpretation, if there's no circle at the top, it indicates six months. If it's missing from the lower part, it indicates three months. If it's missing from the side closer to the nose (for the left eye, the right side of the visual field), this indicates one month. And if it's missing from the side closer to the ear (the left side of the visual field), it indicates two months. This is one way of understanding this technique.

The other method is similar. First, look upward and press gently from below the eye to see whether the circles of light appear. Then look downward and press from above. Next, look toward the nose and press from the outer part of the eye, and finally look toward the ear and press from the inner part.

We are then told to repeat the process, this time with the right eye. If the circles of light are absent from the lower part of the right eye, it means that death will occur after ten days. This is the line that was copied into the *Śiva Svarodaya*. If the circles are absent from the upper part, it means that one will die after five days. If they are absent from the direction of the right ear, the person will die in three days, and if they are absent from the direction of the right nostril, one will die in two days, even if not sick. This, in my view, is one of the most interesting techniques within this "science" of determining the moment of death.

Predictions Based on Eye Circles

Eye	Missing Circle Location	Time Until Death
Left Eye	Lower part	6 months
Left Eye	Upper part	3 months
Left Eye	Direction of nostril (inner)	1 month
Left Eye	Direction of ear (outer)	2 months
Right Eye	Lower part	10 days
Right Eye	Upper part	5 days
Right Eye	Direction of ear (outer)	3 days
Right Eye	Direction of nostril (inner)	2 days

Chāyopāsana: The Shadow Gazing Technique

I believe that the ultimate and most intriguing technique is the final one presented in this chapter, called *Chāyopāsana*, the practice of gazing at the shadow.

The *Śiva Svarodaya* Version

The *Śiva Svarodaya* gives the following instruction for *Chāyopāsana*: "Going alone to a lonely place and keeping the sun at one's back, one should fix the attention on the throat area of one's shadow. Then one should look toward the sky while reciting the mantra *'Hrīṃ Para Brahmaṇena Mahā'* 108 times, after which the form of Śiva is seen.

The practitioner will then see Lord Śiva, whose appearance is like pure crystal and who assumes numerous forms. One who practices this *upāsanā* (technique) for six months becomes a king, and if he continues to practice for two years, he may himself become the creator, destroyer, and all-powerful Lord. Through regular constant practice, the yogi becomes the knower of the three times (past, present & future) and attains absolute bliss. Nothing remains inaccessible to him".

Interpretations of the Vision

If the practitioner or yogī sees in the clear sky the form of Śiva as black-colored, they will undoubtedly die within six months. If Śiva's form appears yellow, the practitioner will suffer from disease; if red, from fear; if blue, from loss; and if multicolored, they will attain success or paranormal powers. If the feet, ankles, and belly are missing from the form of Śiva, the practitioner will meet gradual destruction, and if both arms are missing, they will definitely die. If the left arm is missing, the text says that the wife will die, and if the right arm is missing, a kinsman will die, and within a month, the practitioner will also die.

If the thighs or shoulders are not seen, death will occur within eight days. If no shadow of the form is seen at all, then death is said to occur at that very moment.

In the morning, one is instructed to stand with the sun at their back and concentrate on the shadow. If the fingers and the lips of the shadow are missing, then death is said to be immediate. One who is unable to see their own shadow at all can expect death within a moment. If the ears, shoulders, hands, face, sides, or chest are not visible in the shadow, death is said to come in half a second.

If the shadow appears headless and, at the same time, the person does not know the significance of the different directions—does not know where north and south are in that moment—then they will live only up to six months. This is how the technique is described in the *Śiva Svarodaya.*

The Elaborated Tibetan Version

The Tibetan version of this method, found in the Tibetan Book of the Dead, is more elaborate. It begins with making offerings to the spiritual teacher and to the Three Precious Jewels: the Buddha, the Dharma (his teachings), and the Saṅgha (the spiritual community). Then a torma offering is made—sculpted forms, usually of flour and butter colored with various dyes, are offered to different spirits and entities that might interfere with the process, asking them to leave the practitioner undisturbed.

Preparations and Conditions

The practitioner is then invited to offer multiple prayers and to perform their practice in an isolated place in either the morning or afternoon on the first day of the month, or possibly in the evening or at dawn on the fifteenth lunar day, when the sky is clear, there is no wind, no one can see you, and there are no clouds in the sky. After praying for clear information, the mantra "*Oṃ Āyuṣe Saṃhāra Kiśvare Hūṃ Phaṭ*" is repeated 100 times.

The Practice Procedure

The person should then stand naked and bow down seven times to each of the devas of the ten directions. With the arms extended, the practitioner is instructed to hold in one hand a rosary or another ritual emblem, and then to visualize or inscribe the letter "A" at the heart of their shadow.

Without blinking, practicing what we have learned as trāṭaka, they should gaze steadily at this letter "A" in the shadow until the eyes grow very tired. Then the yogi should look straight up into the cloudless sky, where they are said to see their own form—not the form of Śiva as in the Svarodaya texts, but their own—appearing in the sky.

Interpreting the Aerial Image

Then the text tells us: "One should know then that if the head and body of this image are intact and the image is pale in color; it is an auspicious sign and there will be no obstacles and death will not happen". If the image does not appear, the practitioner is invited to reaffirm their Buddhist vows, sit in the lotus posture with the hands resting in the lap, and then look again. If it still does not appear, the process should be postponed and the shadow observed on a different day.

When the image does appear in the sky, the practitioner is instructed to examine three aspects of it: its completeness, its shape, and its color. While I cannot describe every detail from the Tibetan Book of the Dead, the main points are highlighted below so that you can follow the essence of the practice, and you can always turn to the full text if you wish to go deeper.

Predictions Based on Completeness

If the object you're holding in your hand does not appear in the aerial image, it is said that life may end in seven years. If the right hand is missing, this means one may die after five years; if the left hand is missing, after three years. If the right leg is missing below the knee, one may die after two years, and if it's the left leg, after one year.

If the right side of the head is missing, one may die after nine months. If the left side is missing, after seven months. If the head is missing above the neck, death may occur after five months, and if both head and neck are missing, only three months are said to remain.

If the upper trunk is missing, death may come after two months. If the lower trunk is missing, after one month. If the entire right side of the body is missing, one may die in 29 days, and if the left side is missing, in 21 days.

Missing Body Part	Time Until Death
Object in hand	7 years
Right hand	5 years
Left hand	3 years
Right leg (below knee)	2 years
Left leg (below knee)	1 year
Right part of head	9 months
Left part of head	7 months
Head above neck	5 months
Head and neck	3 months
Upper trunk	2 months
Lower trunk	1 month
Entire right side	29 days
Entire left side	21 days

Predictions Based on Shape

After examining the completeness of the image, the next step is to look carefully at the shape of the body.

If the image appears square, it is said that one may die after five months; if it is round, after four. If it is semicircular, death is predicted after three months. If oblong, after two. And if triangular, after one month. If it resembles a bundled corpse, the indication is a month and a half, and if it appears upside down, ten days.

The text adds that, except for these last three shapes: bundled like a corpse, triangular, or upside down, that death can in principle be averted. If any of those three appear, however, then death is considered definite.

Shape	Time Until Death
Square	5 months
Round	4 months
Semicircular	3 months
Oblong	2 months
Triangle	1 month
Bundled corpse	1.5 months
Upside down	10 days

Predictions Based on Color

Finally, color and the way the image fades are each said to carry specific meanings. The practitioner is instructed to note the color that the "shadow in the sky" takes on after gazing at the shadow and then shifting the gaze upward, and to read further meanings from that coloration. The Tibetan text summarizes these colors and patterns in a series of indications:

If the image is white and fades from the center, this is said to indicate an imbalance of the water element. If it is black colored and fades from the side, it suggests issues with various female forces in the body. If it is red colored and fades from the left, this is interpreted as the influence of violent spirits or as a sign that wounds and diseases may appear soon.

If it is yellow and fades from the head, this again points to interference from the water element or from water spirits. If it is blue and fades from the legs, it is said that the water elements—and specifically lake-dwelling spirits—are affecting the person. If the image is hazy and diffuse, it indicates various female spirits attacking the person. If it appears yellowish and uneven, it points to issues with the earth element. If it is garish, irregular, and variegated, this means that all eight classes of spirits have attacked the individual. This is the gist of what is given in the Tibetan Book of the Dead.

Color & Fading Pattern	Indication
White, fades from center	Imbalance of water element
Black, fades from side	Issues with various female forces in the body
Red, fades from left	Influence of violent spirits, or wounds and diseases coming soon
Yellow, fades from head	Interference from water element or water spirits
Blue, fades from legs	Influence of water elements and lake-dwelling spirits
Hazy and diffuse	Various female spirits attacking the person
Yellowish and uneven	Issues with element of earth
Garish, irregular, variegated	All eight classes of spirits have attacked the individual

What to do with These Predictions

At this point, a natural question arises: what should you do if such a practice suggests that you have only a limited time to live? Both the *Śiva Svarodaya* and the Tibetan Book of the Dead are clear that these signs are not final verdicts. A sign indicating that death may occur in six months is not a fixed sentence. It's a call to recognize that something unhealthy might be going in your system and that it needs attention.

In Tibetan and Indian traditions, this would traditionally be addressed through prayers, mantras, and various ritual practices. If you feel drawn to that path, I invite you to explore the Tibetan Book of the Dead for more detail.

For many modern practitioners, though, it can be more helpful to treat these indications as invitations to care for our health: to support the body, to go for checkups, to consult appropriate medical professionals, and to take practical steps to bring life back toward balance.

Closing Reflections

Once again, none of these signs have actually been proven or researched in any modern, systematic way, and they are presented here simply at face value. Hopefully you have found them interesting.

If you experiment with any of these practices and feel you need guidance in how to relate to the results, or if you would like a deeper explanation of the rites and techniques that are said to alleviate these issues, you are warmly invited to write to me, and I will support you as much as possible.

I hope you found this interesting, though it is understandable if you find all of this a little strange. It bears repeating that none of it has been empirically proven. Still, the hope is that you have found it at least enjoyable and possibly instructive.

The Svarodaya literature contains one final dimension still to explore: using these principles for divination and for predicting outcomes for those who seek guidance.

Chapter 27

Divination Through Svara: Applying Svara Wisdom to Astrology, Tarot, and Divination

In this book, I chose to focus on what feels like the most relevant and engaging aspect of the Svarodaya literature for us today: using Svara Yoga as an art of right timing. This means aligning our actions with both our internal cycles and the cycles of nature, so that we can live more harmoniously and allow our efforts to bear fruit with greater ease, letting life and prosperity flow more naturally.

Along the way, I have also touched on some of the more esoteric aspects of this teaching, such as the signs of death and methods for family planning. One subject has been left aside until now, and this chapter turns to it directly: the subject of divination.

When looking carefully at the *Śiva Svarodaya*, it becomes clear that a significant part of the text is written specifically with astrologers in mind, astrologers who are consulted by clients. Moreover, if we then look at the second main text of this tradition, the *Svara cintāmaṇi*, we see that it is largely devoted to advice for professional divinators and astrologers on how to respond to the questions of clients who come seeking guidance about future events.

The Three-Fold Observation Method

In general, the Svara Śāstra says that when we act as a professional astrologer, palm reader, divinator, or any similar guide whom people approach with questions about their future karma, there are a few key observations to make when a questioner—or a messenger on their behalf—arrives.

First, notice from which direction the questioner is arriving and where they sit when they ask their question. Second, observe which svara is active in you—the diviner—at the exact moment the question is asked. Finally, recognize which element is arising within you at the same moment.

By combining these three factors, and using the keys provided in the Svarodaya literature, it is said that one can begin to answer at least some of the questions posed in a more attuned and insightful way.

Simple Divination Examples

Starting with a very simple case: when a question is asked about someone who has gone away, the texts give the following guidelines:

Active Element(s)	Prediction
Earth or Water	The person is enjoying a contented life, good health, the love of others, entertainment, victory, and pleasure
Fire or Wind	The person is suffering from fever with shivering, or from excessive sleep

Imagine yourself as the astrologer: someone comes to ask about a person who has left. You observe your svara, recognize that the active element is either earth or water, and answer accordingly.

A slightly more subtle example: if a messenger speaks about a desire at the time of your inhalation, that desire will be fulfilled. If they speak at the time of exhalation, it will not. Here the astrologer waits for the person asking the question and maintains a quiet awareness of the breath, without forcing or changing it. If, while the messenger is describing a desire, the astrologer notices that a natural inhalation is taking place, this is read as a sign that the desire will come to fruition.

Complex Divination: War and Conflict

The indications become more complex with questions about war or conflict. When the lunar svara is flowing, the person whose name is simple and common, or contains an even number of letters, gains victory. However, if the questioner stands or sits on the right side, then the one whose name is unusual or has an odd number of letters is victorious.

Another verse says: "If the lunar svara flows while questioning, then there will be a compromise. If the solar svara flows, then know that there will be war".

The Kalottara (1300, 8.154) adds that if Iḍā (the lunar flow) is active during rituals performed to destroy an enemy, victory is predicted within ten days.

The Structure of the Svara cintāmaṇi

While the *Śiva Svarodaya* is not particularly organized (as can be seen from the examples above), the *Svara cintāmaṇi* is divided into clear chapters, each dedicated to a specific kind of question. These include topics such as taking baths, water and food, sickness, war, rain, grains and agriculture, hunting, bad dreams, and more.

Agricultural and Economic Predictions

Vegetation and Crops

As one example, when the query concerns the growth of vegetation and if the lunar nāḍī is operating, the text says that there will be growth. If the solar nāḍī is operating instead, the prediction is destruction. If the lunar nāḍī is flowing fully, there will be abundant growth of all grains, but if the air moves fast, it is said that the harvest will be carried off by thieves.

If the Jala Tattva (water) joins the Agni Tattva (fire) in the lunar nāḍī at the time of a question about grains and agriculture, it indicates modest or limited growth. If the situation is reversed and Agni joins Jala—fire entering into water—there is said to be danger from fire.

Grain Prices

When someone asks specifically about the price of grains, the svara of the astrologer is used directly:

Active Nostril in the Astrologer	Prediction
Left nostril	Prices will be high
Right nostril	Prices will be low
Equal breath between both	Grains will be taken by the government

Annual Predictions: The Solar Year Transition

The *Śiva Svarodaya* also instructs the astrologer to observe which tattva is arising at the exact moment when the solar year begins—when the sun transitions into the sign of Aries. The key idea is to locate the precise transition and then recognize which element is active in that moment.

The rising and setting of the tattvas follows the earth's rotation around its own axis (sunrise and sunset), whereas the movement of the sun into different constellations follows the earth's revolution around the sun. These are different cycles, which means that even if you are fully aligned with natural rhythms, the elemental pattern at that Aries transition may be quite distinct. By observing the tattva that arises at that moment, the astrologer is said to receive a broad prediction for the entire year.

Generally speaking the *Śiva Svarodaya* says the following: "When the earth or water element is prominent, the days, the months and the whole year will be prosperous and hold good news. If the ether, air or fire element is present, the condition will be bad". In details the Elemental predictions are shown the table below

Element at Solar Transition	Annual Prediction
Earth	Abundant food, prosperity, good crops, plentiful rain, and happiness
Water	Sufficient rains, abundance of food, freedom from disease, prosperity, and rich crops
Fire	Famine, destruction, and scanty rainfall
Air	Trouble, calamity, fear, and various natural disasters
Ether	Desolation due to scanty crops and lack of prosperity

As you can see, this material is aimed mainly at astrologers who advise rulers and decision-makers about global events that affect whole regions and countries.

Predictions About Disease

Along with these large-scale readings, some passages are directed toward individual concerns, such as questions about diseases, where the text indicates such things as:

Condition	Prediction
Messenger approaches from the closed-nostril side and sits on the flowing-nostril side	The sick person will survive, even if in a coma
Questioner asks while sitting on the side of the active svara	The patient, though suffering from several diseases, will survive
Svara flows downwards (water element) at the time of questioning	The patient will recover
Svara flows upwards (fire element) at the time of questioning	The patient will certainly arrive at the realm of Yama, the lord of death

Put simply, an approach that "moves toward" the open nostril and a downward-flowing svara is considered a positive sign, whereas an upward-flowing svara in this context is read as an indication of approaching death.

The *Śiva Svarodaya* and, especially, the *Svara cintāmaṇi*, were written primarily for court astrologers and spiritual advisors, whose role was to counsel rulers on matters of state, agriculture, warfare, and cosmic timing. The elaborate systems for answering questions about grain prices, rainfall, and military outcomes reflect a world in which breath-reading function as a tool of statecraft.

Few modern readers—aside from those of you who are practicing astrologers—will use Svara Yoga in this way to answer clients' questions. Yet the underlying skills can still support daily life whenever someone approaches you with a request. Learning to sense the outcome of a request based on the relationship between your breath and the person in front of you does have modern equivalents, and I invite you to explore how this might apply in your life.

Dream Interpretation according to the Kalottara Tantra

Since the Kalottara Tantra has never before been translated, this section shares as much as possible from the original verses, with references to their location. In chapter 8 of the 1300-verse Kalottara, beginning at verse 104, we are taught how to distinguish dreams that are genuinely divinatory from those that are not. The night (beginning at sunset) is divided into segments, each with its own dream quality.

Dreams in the first part of the night are said to arise from the day's events:

> "A dream that arises from mental impressions is said to be emotionally imagined. Whatever was done during the day, including mantric acts, appears in it".

In the second part of the night, governed by Jayā nāḍī, confusing dreams arise from the vāta element:

> "One rooted in emotion or bhāva perceives a subtle thread during the first night quarter. When Jayā nāḍī is flowing, a vāta-related dream may occur, O Skanda".

The third portion of the night is ruled by pitta and brings clearer dreams—though even here, confused dreams may still echo the day's events. The fourth portion is associated with kappha and brings calm, dense, or heavy dreams:

> "In the third portion of the night, during Vijayā nāḍī's flow, the pitta-based dream arises. In the last quarter, dreams are of the kapha type (calm, dense, or heavy)".

The very last part of the night is described as containing mixed-dosha dreams:

> "In the last part of the night, mixed-doṣa dreams (sannipāta) occur uninterruptedly, Until dawn, this state is referred to as the end of uṣā (twilight)".

Of prophetic dreams, the text says:

> "The one who perceives mixed or false dreams due to vāta, etc., Should know that future outcomes are of two types: auspicious and inauspicious".

Finally, the Kalottara offers a simple key linking dreams and svara:

> "Dreams that occur during Iḍā flow bring auspicious outcomes; otherwise, the result is the reverse. This is because of all the nāḍīs, the Iḍā carries the most pure and beneficial current".
>
> (Kalottara 1300, 8.104-109)

PART VI:
THE SVARA TRANSCENDED

Chapter 28
Astrological Purification in the Kalachakra Tantra

While Svara Yoga, as explored so far, focuses mainly on living in harmony with the cycles of nature, the deeper aim of yoga has always been much higher: to either master nature or to transcend it altogether. This transcending is what is called liberation.

Liberation means freedom—freedom from the influence of the internal movements of prāṇa that stir the suffering mind, as well as from the external forces of nature that shape those movements. For as long as we are controlled by any force, internal or external, we are not truly free. Ultimately, as this section will show, the teachings point toward attaining freedom from even time itself.

One way to understand these external influences is to compare Eastern and Western astrology. Western astrology focuses mainly on how the planets—what could be called the "external svara"—influence the personality of the individual. A horoscope is intended to show how each planet, its position, and its relationship to other planets at the time of birth affect the individual and shapes their personality.

By contrast, the Indian and Tibetan astrological systems describe how the particular arrangement of planets at birth determines the karma that will affect, or even afflict, the person. In other words, it predicts the unfolding events of one's life and, ultimately, the path towards enlightenment, because the very reason one is not yet enlightened is karma itself. To become enlightened, the yogi must “burn” or “transcend” their karma.

Karma, in our context, means an “impulse of energy” that shapes both external and internal events—from the movement of the planets, to natural calamities and political developments, and from the cycles of the body to the cycles of the mind.

More advanced teachings that make use of svara do not only show how to harmonize our inner rhythms with the rhythms of nature; they also point toward completely transcending these rhythms. This means becoming free of the astrological influences that determine our karma and external events, free from any sense of predetermined destiny, and even free from time itself.

If this idea is applied to the way astrology is usually seen in the West, it would amount to becoming free from your astrological sign. Your horoscope would no longer define you; even if you once wished you had been born under a different sign, you would now be free to choose how to be in the world, regardless of what your chart says.

Kalachakra - Inner, Outer, and Alternative

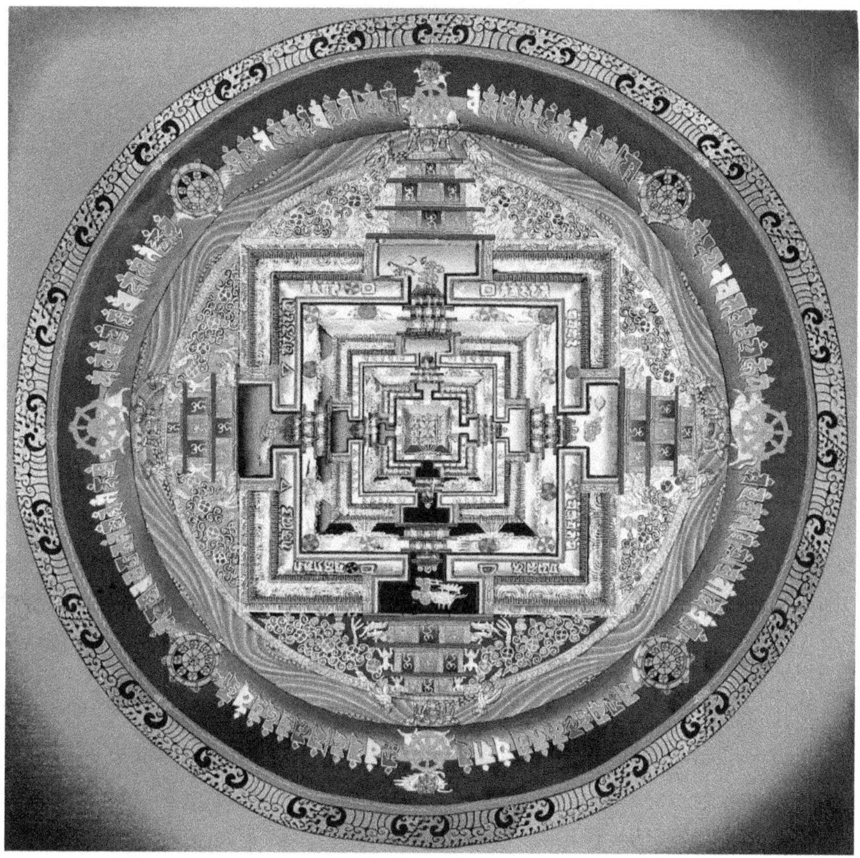

The teaching on transcending astrological influences and astrological time appears in its clearest form in the Tibetan *Kālacakra Tantra*, the 11th-century tantra of the "wheel of time" or "the cycles of time". In January 2006, I participated in the Kālacakra Initiation held by H. H. Tenzin Gyatso, the 14th Dalai Lama, but it took me over a decade to begin studying it in depth, and another decade before I recognized its connection with the teachings of Svara Yoga.

I am not a Vajra Master in the Tibetan lineage—someone authorized to give this initiation—but since the Dalai Lama has declared that the time of secrecy around the tantras is over and that these teachings can be shared openly, I share the underlying theory of this system here. Should you decide you wish to practice it, I invite you to seek initiation and practical guidance from a qualified teacher.

The *Kālacakra Tantra* teaches of three interconnected cycles: the external cycles of the celestial objects, the internal cycles of breath and mind, and the "alternative" cycle, which is the Kālacakra path itself, showing how to overcome the first two.

The external cycles include the vast rhythms through which our universe passes through: the creation and destruction of eons corresponding to the big bang, the formation and rotation of galaxies, and the cycles of sun and planets, earth and moon. The internal cycles include those of our physical body—menstruation, hormones, hunger and thirst, tiredness and wakefulness—as well as the great arc of birth, aging, and death, and even the smaller cycles of inhalation and exhalation, including the subtle shifts of svara from left to right, and through the elements within each breath.

The Kālacakra explains the connection between these inner and outer cycles in a way that differs from the usual idea that planets affect us through subtle mechanisms or the projection of "energies" across space. Instead, both inner and outer cycles are said to be aligned expressions of karma itself. Other traditions describe the planets (in Sanskrit *grahas,* "seizers") as power that capture the individual within the cycles of karma and act as the "lackeys of time", exerting time's karmic influence through the "ravages" of change, decay, and fate. The Kālacakra reverses this: universal cycles themselves arise from karma rather than creating it. The planets are governed by the collective karma of humanity, and since collective karma is made up of the karmas of individuals, the internal and external cycles mirror one another.

The "alternative" Kālacakra is so named because it provides an alternative cycle, structured in the same way as the external and internal cycles, but designed to help the practitioner overcome them and become free of their hold. It offers a systematic method for purifying all the "influences" that the cycles of time exert on a being, and it does so in two main stages or phases of practice.

Purification through visualization of the Generation stage

The first practice of purification is known as the *Kalachakra Generation Stage*. Here, the practitioner is supposed to visualize the Kālacakra mandala so intensely that they become fully identified and one with it, as if merging into its form and energy.

The Kālacakra mandala is a symbolic representation of all the forces that make up the human being and nature, including all the forces acting on behalf of time in accordance with karma.

These forces are depicted by as 722 deities that inhabit the mandala. The easiest way to understand what a deity means in this context is to reflect on the word 'divine'. What is a "divinely" tasty cake? It's a cake whose flavor has been refined and purified until it becomes the ultimate, best taste.

In the same way, each deity is a personified, symbolic representation of the most purified essence of what it stands for: the deity of earth is the symbol of the earth in its purest form, and the deity of sight is our capacity to see clearly and without distortion.

Within the mandala, there are symbolic representations of the elements of nature, the elements of the mind, the senses, the actions, and all the different aspects of time: the 12 months of the year, the 30 lunar days, day and night, the two halves of the year, the seasons, down to each and every moment. All of these are also linked to the various energy channels in the body and the channels in the chakras, through which the karmic winds flow and shape our state of mind.

From this whole network of influences, the 12 zodiacal signs are especially important, because Kālacakra connects them with the 12 steps of dependent origination. These 12 steps of dependent origination are the Buddha's explanation of how the endless samsaric cycle of suffering continuously unfolds and repeats itself throughout our lives.

The 12 links of dependent origination

The 12 links of dependent origination are described in the Kalachakra as an inner cycle that keeps the wheel of samsaric suffering turning.

1. Ignorance (avidyā) – not seeing reality correctly, *leading to...*
2. Formations (saṃskāra) – karmic impulses and actions conditioned by ignorance, *leading to...*
3. Consciousness (vijñāna) – a "loaded" stream of awareness carrying karmic tendencies, *leading to...*
4. Name-and-form (nāmarūpa) – mentality and materiality, *leading to...*
5. Six sense bases (ṣaḍāyatana) – eye, ear, nose, tongue, body, and mind, *leading to...*
6. Contact (sparśa) – the meeting of sense base, object, and consciousness, *leading to...*
7. Feeling (vedanā) – the pleasant, unpleasant, or neutral tones of experience, *leading to...*
8. Craving (tṛṣṇā "thirst") – grasping at pleasant experiences and pushing away unpleasant ones, a crucial point for activating karma (Kalachakra talks often highlight links 8–10 at death) , *leading to...*
9. Clinging (upādāna) – "obtainer" attitudes such as fixation and possessiveness, *leading to...*
10. Becoming (bhava) – karmic becoming, the momentum ripening toward rebirth, *leading to...*
11. Birth (jāti) – the arising of a new life stream, *leading to...*
12. Aging-and-death (jarā-maraṇa) – the decline and ending of that stream, the endpoint of the suffering aggregate

The Kālacakra connects these 12 links with the 12 zodiacal signs, starting with Ignorance in Capricorn, so that regardless of the calendar month you are born in, there is an inner cycle that begins at birth with Capricorn. These links are said to be directly purified by the Kalachakra deity mother-and-father pair in the center of the mandala.

The purification through the Yogas of the completion stage

According to the Kalachakra teachings, the objective cause of suffering is time itself. The Buddha taught that everything in this universe that is subject to time is suffering; this is his second of the Four Noble Truths about our world.

According to the buddha life brings two broad types of experiences: painful experiences that we clearly do not want, and joyful experiences that we usually cherish. Why are even joyful experiences considered suffering? Because, as the Buddha's first Noble Truth points out, everything in our world is transient—since all good things must eventually pass, time itself turns even joy into a subtle form of suffering. Without time there can be no unfolding of the 12 links of dependent origination, and without those links, there is no suffering.

Time is therefore the external or objective cause of suffering, while the internal or subjective cause is the mind. If the mind is enlightened and does not cling to things that arise and pass in time, it can transcend this suffering. Later chapters will describe how this enlightened mind is actually a kind of "no-mind" that exists beyond time, and how stopping "internal time" is another way to transcend the svara.

Many yogic sources state that "wherever prana goes, the mind goes". This teaching explains that the mind is driven by the inner winds of the body—the subtle movements of prana—which are themselves controlled by karma, the karmic winds.

According to the Kālacakra teachings, there are 21,600 karmic winds that manifest as the 21,600 breaths a person is said to have in a single day. Each day, the same 21,600 karmic winds reappear in this repeating daily cycle.

Of these 21,000, about 20,925 are considered karmic breaths and flow through the side channels of the body, and 675 are considered breaths of wisdom that flow through the central channel. These 675 breaths of wisdom correspond to the spontaneous moments, each day, when the svaras become equal.

In what is called the Completion Stage, the yogi is supposed to go through 21,600 instances of generating bliss through various techniques. An "instance" here means a period of time that can be as short as a single moment or as long as an entire meditation session.

Each moment of unchanging, blissful awareness burns off one of the 21,600 karmic winds and, with it, one portion of the deeply ingrained habits created by karma. Once a particular karmic wind is purified, the breath associated with it no longer flows through the side channels; instead, it flows only through the central channel. When this shift happens, karma loses its power over the practitioner. The yogi has overcome the karmic forces that used to drive the winds into the side channels and from there into all the different channels of the body. When the winds no longer move through the 72,000 nadis, the mind has nothing to ride on and cannot be carried anywhere. In that condition, no suffering can be experienced; one is no longer affected by inner forces or by the forces of nature that once drove those inner forces. Once the yogi has completed all 21,600 moments—accomplished in 12 stages connected with the 6 chakras, the 12 zodiac signs, and the rising of energy through the spine—their gross and subtle bodies dissolve. They then reach the enlightened, liberated state of a Buddha. From that point on, the yogi is completely free, no longer bound to the influences of karma, the stars, or the svara—free from both the external cycles and the internal cycles as one.

Chapter 29
Speeding Up Evolution Through Svara: The Cycles in Kriya Yoga & the Tantras

In his 1946 book *Autobiography of a Yogi*, Paramahamsa Yogananda, the great teacher of Kriya Yoga in the West, reports that his teacher Sri Yukteshwar used to say that, “Kriya Yoga is an instrument through which human evolution can be quickened”. In chapter 26 of the book, devoted to explaining the science of Kriya Yoga, Yogananda describes the mechanism behind this statement.

> “The Kriya Yogi mentally directs his life energy to revolve, upward and downward, around the six spinal centers (medullary, cervical, dorsal, lumbar, sacral, and coccygeal plexuses) which correspond to the twelve astral signs of the zodiac, the symbolic Cosmic Man. One-half minute of revolution of energy around the sensitive spinal cord of man effects subtle progress in his evolution; that half-minute of Kriya equals one year of natural spiritual unfoldment.
>
> The astral system of a human being, with six (twelve by polarity) inner constellations revolving around the sun of the omniscient spiritual eye, is interrelated with the physical sun and the twelve zodiacal signs. All men are thus affected by an inner and an outer universe. The ancient rishis discovered that man's earthly and heavenly environment, in twelve-year cycles, push him

> forward on his natural path. The scriptures aver that man requires a million years of normal, diseaseless evolution to perfect his human brain sufficiently to express cosmic consciousness.
>
> One thousand Kriya practiced in eight hours gives the yogi, in one day, the equivalent of one thousand years of natural evolution: 365,000 years of evolution in one year. In three years, a Kriya Yogi can thus accomplish by intelligent self-effort the same result which nature brings to pass in a million years".
>
> From *Autobiography of a Yogi* (1946 edition, public-domain text via Project Gutenberg)

Though Yogananda claimed that this teaching was lost for millennia and only revived by his adi-guru Babaji, who instructed it to Lahiri Mahasaya (the teacher of Sri Yukteshwar), this core teaching actually appears in many traditional tantric writings.

The earliest known form of this teaching seems to be from the 6th-7th century *Kalottara Tantra*, later elaborated in the 7th *century Svaccanda Tantra*, and then explained in great detail in the 10th century by the Kashmiri master Abhinavagupta in his authoritative expositions of tantra, the *Tantraloka*.

The underlying principle shared by all these sources is that the normal evolution that unfolds though the hamsa mantra—constantly being emitted by the breath—can be hastened when its link to the cosmic cycles is brought into awareness and consciously meditated upon.

The *Kalottara Tantra*, the earliest of these texts, teaches: "One revolution of Nāda is equal to countless external years" and "By knowing this wheel (of time), one perceives time as motion within breath. He who turns it inward crosses the course of years and aeons".

Abhinavagupta introduces this teaching with particular beauty and precision in chapter 6 of his *Tantraloka*. In verses 92-98, he explains the meaning and function behind this doctrine in a way that has shaped much of the later tantric understanding of breath, sound, and time:

> "A whole day and night may last a moment—or a moment may extend for an age (kalpa). The length of a moment depends on the clarity of consciousness. For ordinary perception it's a fleeting instant, but for yogic God-consciousness it expands to timelessness. Hence one breath may contain months and years".

Why does this form of meditation burn more karma and speed up our evolution? Another way of looking at it is to say that evolution happens through the passing of time (which is marked by the breath), and time brings all the events in our life that drive us to grow and evolve. When we sharpen the mind and recognize the link between the inner cycle of inhale and exhale and all the parallel cycles in nature, our subjective sense of time slows down. This can allow us to experience the equivalent of even a year's worth of evolution in a single breath.

The sharpening of the mind and slowing of time may occur through direct perception of the timeless nature of our consciousness, through increased concentration, or through the power of creative imagination (*bhāvanā*). This kind of imagination is not mere daydreaming; but actually brings into being what is imagined.

Thus all these sources point to the same insight: the breath mirrors the cosmic rhythm of creation and dissolution, and all cosmic cycles of time manifest themselves in the in-breath and out-breath. Each breath thus model of a 24-hour day in miniature.

The cycle of the day

First, we have the cycle of the day: each breath contains a sunrise, midday, sunset, and midnight within it. In traditional measurements, the breath in meditation, from the heart to the "end of the twelve", is said to travel a distance of 36 *aṅgula* (finger-widths), where the "end of twelve" can mean either 12 fingers beyond the nostrils or 12 fingers above the crown.

In reality, the breath can be sensed as moving deeper and lower in the body than the chest—down to the navel in some meditations, the root, or even as far as the big toes. But movement below the heart (or below the navel in some traditions) is usually unconscious, which is why most meditations describe the breath as moving from the center of the chest to the space outside.

In this model, inhalation begins at the end of the twelve and corresponds to the *iḍā*, the lunar, cooling night time. As the air reaches the uvula at the back of the mouth, it is equated with the middle of the night, and dawn—the transition between night and day—happens in the heart (or the navel, in some readings). Then night turns into day as the air is exhaled. The breath reaches "midday" again at the uvula, and dusk—the transition between day and night—at the end of the twelve.

In this way, every 30-breath cycles form an inner month, while 21,600 breaths (one full day and night of breathing) equal an outer year. Yet each single breath also holds within it all the other cycles of time.

The lunar month cycle

The same breath can be read as the monthly cycle of the moon. Inhalation is equated with *Śukla Pakṣa*, the waxing moon: as the light increases, starting from the new moon at the "end of 12" when the lungs are empty, and culminating in the full moon when the lungs are full and the breath rests at the heart. Exhale (*Kṛṣṇa Pakṣa*) is linked with the waning moon, as the moon "empties" together with the air leaving the lungs and the light gradually diminishes.

You may visualize inhalation as light emerging from darkness (moon waxing), and exhalation as light dissolving back into darkness (moon waning).

The Solar Half-Year Cycles: Uttarāyaṇa and Dakṣiṇāyana:

Exhalation is equated with Uttarāyaṇa, the sun's northward course, the "day" of the breath. It begins at the Winter Solstice (Capricorn) in the heart, as the outward *prāṇa* starts to ascend, passes the Spring Equinox at the palate/uvula, and ends at the Summer Solstice (Gemini/Cancer) at the *dvādaśānta* (the "end of twelve"), when the breath is fully expanded outward.

Inhalation (Dakṣiṇāyana) is linked with the sun's southward course, the "night" of the breath. It begins at the Summer Solstice as the *apāna* is drawn back inward, passes the Autumn Equinox at the palate, and completes its journey by dissolving back into the heart at the Winter Solstice (Sagittarius/Capricorn).

The Zodiac within Breath

Next, the 12 solar months (connected with 12 Rudras) or the changing of the zodiac can be mapped into the breath. The 12 *rāśi*, or zodiac signs, are spread across the 360 degrees of the sky and also across the 72 aṅgulas of the breath (36 on inhale and 36 on exhale). This means that every six finger-breadths of movement of air, starting from the heart, the inner "sun" abides in a different sign of the zodiac. The journey begins with Capricorn in the heart and moves all the way to Gemini at the *dvādaśānta*, then returns from Cancer back through the signs until it reaches Sagittarius and Capricorn back in the heart.

The process of superimposing the year onto the breath becomes even more significant when we understand it a spiritual allegory. An entire lifetime that is encoded into this subtle journey of prāṇa with each breath:

Sign	Stage (Skt.)	Translation	The Spiritual Meaning
Aries	Garbha-daśā	Embryonic Stage	The "seed" state. The initial conception where potential is hidden in the womb of the mind.
Taurus	Icchā	Will / Desire	The impulse to take form. The vague idea becomes a solid desire to exist.
Gemini	Abhilāṣa	Longing / Aspiration	The desire seeks expression and communication. The "plan" begins to take shape in words.
Cancer	Prasava-sannidhi	Impending Birth	The stage of the "shell". The project is fully formed but still protected/ nurtured within.
Leo	Prasava	Birth / Manifestation	The "I am" moment. The energy steps out of the womb and into the light of day.
Virgo	Vikāsa	Expansion / Analysis	The refinement phase. Sorting, organizing, and perfecting the details of the life or work.
Libra	Prabhā	Radiance / Reflection	The "mirror" stage. Recognizing oneself through others and finding balance in relationships.
Scorpio	Viṣaya	Sensory Depth	Intense experience. Digging deep into the "matter" of life, often involving crisis and transformation.
Sagittarius	Pratibhā	Spiritual Genius	The flash of insight. Moving beyond the personal to see the universal truth or higher law.
Capricorn	Sthiti	Consolidation	Reaching the peak. Establishing a legacy, a structure, or a physical foundation in the world.
Aquarius	Upalabdhi	Realization	Attainment of the goal. Distributing the "water" of knowledge to the collective; service.
Pisces	Laya	Dissolution	Merging back into the source. The completion of the cycle and the return to the void.

When awareness follows this inner zodiac fully, the yogin experiences birth, growth, decay, and reabsorption into the divine womb all within a single breath, allowing the experiencing of a karmic evolution equivalent to an entire lifetime.

The Great Cycles of Jupiter and Saturn

Next come the great cycles of Jupiter and Saturn (12 and 60 years).

Jupiter completes one round of the zodiac in 12 years, while Saturn takes about 29½ years, and their conjunction in the same zodiac repeat every 60 years (21,600 days)—the same number as daily breaths.

"Thus 21,600 breaths in a day equal the 21,600 days in a 60-year cycle—microcosm and macrocosm united". The *Svacchanda Tantra* takes this proportion and projects it into each breath, making every exhalation-inhalation a miniature cosmic conjunction.

Even longer cycles can also be superimposed onto the breath. Indian cosmology is full of vast cycles:

The 4 yugas, an immense cycle of the rise and fall of humanity, moving from an age of truth through successive degenerations into the dark age called "Kālī Yuga"—the age said to be now—lasts 4,320,000 years.

- A *Manvatara*, the lifespan of a human species, said to last 71 cycles of yugas (4.32 million x 71).
- A Kalpa, the lifespan of the universe in its manifest form, is made of 14 *Manvataras.*
- A *Mahā-Kalpa*, the lifespan of the creator of the universe, who creates and reabsorbs the universe hundreds of times.
- A Śrīkaṇṭha lifespan, 100 times that again, leading up to a "*Mahā-Pralaya*" (Great Dissolution), the full process of manifesting and dissolving all universes.

The breath of the universe

Projecting the creation, maintenance, and dissolution of the universe onto the breath is understood, in the tantric tradition, to happen through the unfolding of mantras—specifically the phonemes of the Sanskrit alphabet. The cosmic process is described in terms of the breath as follows: exhalation is the process of creation, beginning in the heart with the Sanskrit vowels rising from the heart to the throat.

"A... Ā... I... Ī... U... Ū... Ṛ... Ṝ... Ḷ... Ḹ... E... Ai... O... Au... Aṁ... Aḥ..."

From the throat, sound deepens into the gutturals:

"Ka, Kha, Ga, Gha, Ṅa".

As the breath flows to the palate, sound becomes lighter in the palatals:

"Ca, Cha, Ja, Jha, Ña".

Higher still, at the roof of the mouth, feel the crisp resonance of the cerebrals:

"Ṭa, Ṭha, Ḍa, Ḍha, Ṇa".

Then, near the teeth ridge, the air strikes gently, producing the dentals:

"Ta, Tha, Da, Dha, Na".

At the lips, as the breath prepares to leave the body, sense the rounded softness of the labials:

"Pa, Pha, Ba, Bha, Ma".

As the breath finally leaves the lips, the four semi-vowels arise:

"Ya, Ra, La, Va"

And at the very threshold where air escapes into the world and creation becomes fully objective, the last four letters emerge:

"Śa, Ṣa, Sa, Ha"

Inhalation traces the return journey, the course of Śakti back to her source, undoing creation by reversing this sequence:

"Ha Sa Ṣa Śa Va La Ra Ya
Ma Bha Ba Pha P
Nā Dha Da Tha Ta
Ṇa Ḍha Ḍa Ṭha Ṭa
Ña Jha Ja Cha Ca
Ṅa Gha Ga Kha Ka

Aḥ Aṁ Au O Ai E Ị̄ Ḷ Ṝ Ṛ Ū U Ī I Ā A".

Mystical time dilation

Time feels different in different states of mind. When lovers are fully present with one another, hours can pass like minutes, while ruminating on suffering can make each moment drag at a snail's pace.

In meditation, as thoughts grow quieter, the perception of time naturally slows down. The simple 4-second span of an ordinary breath can then be subjectively experienced as containing all the time cycles described above, allowing one, it is said, to "live" many lives inwardly and evolve from them as if they were real.

When meditation reaches its culmination in the thought-free experience of Samadhi, this mythical time dilation reaches its peak. What remains is timeless consciousness itself—the subject of our next chapter.

Chapter 30

The Timeless moment of the Kalottara Tantra & in Abhinavaguptas Tantraloka

कालः पचति भूतानि सर्वाण्येवात्मनात्मनि
यस्मिस्तु पच्यते कालस्तं न वेदेह कश्चन ॥ २५ ॥

"Time cooks all beings within the Self; the one in whom Time itself is cooked—none here knows".

- Mahabharata Shanti parvan Verse 12.231.25

If we take the experience of time dilation to its ultimate, we arrive at the liberating state beyond time. When time ceases, nothing remains but pure presence, beyond past and future.

In timelessness, nothing "happens". It is a liberated moment of absolute freedom, untouched by any karmic limitation. Karma, can only function within time—where there is timelessness, there is no coming or going, no change, no action, and thus no karma. To be free of time is to be free of karma, of influence, of suffering—to be truly liberated.

There is freedom from suffering because there is no mind left that can suffer. The mind exists only time: in the past, ruminating over what was lost and still desired, or in the future, fearing what might come.

The yogic tradition of Patanjala Yoga teaches entry into this timeless moment—Samadhi—through meditation: "yogaś citta-vṛtti-nirodhaḥ", yoga is the cessation of the fluctuations of the mind, which is essentially a description of a timeless moment.

While Patañjali emphasizes progressive stages of concentration and meditation, the tantric teachings of Svara Yoga offer a more esoteric way of "falling between the cracks of time". Just as Svara Yoga's teachings on external cycles reveal the right moments to act for worldly results, they also point to specific astrological moments when external influences pause and consciousness can rest in the śūnya, the state of nothingness and no-time. In fact, knowledge of outer moments that support transcendence long predates the detailed teachings on the inner svara.

Already in the early Vedic tradition, practitioners were instructed to perform their household spiritual duties at the four transitional moments of the day, the four *sandhyā-s* ("twilights" or "junctions").

Phase	Sanskrit name	Modern equivalent	Function
1. Prātaḥ-sandhyā	Morning juncture	**Dawn → Sunrise**	Meeting of night and day—ritual *gāyatrī-japa*, *Agnihotra*
2. Madhyāhna-sandhyā	Midday juncture	**Noon**	Balance of rising & setting halves of the sun— *Sūrya-upasthāna*
3. Sāyam-sandhyā	Evening juncture	**Sunset → Dusk**	Meeting of day and night—evening *Agnihotra*, *Sāvitrī-japa*
4. Ardha-rātri-sandhyā	Midnight juncture	**Midnight**	Meeting of waning and waxing halves of night —introspective, used in Soma & Atharvanic rites

These are considered the daily "equinoxes" (viṣuva-s)—moments when opposing temporal or solar forces are perfectly poised, allowing things beyond the ordinary to occur. In the tantras, such junctions are described as especially conducive to meditation and awakening.

Beyond these daily thresholds, the moments of the new and full moon are also regarded as auspicious, as are all lunar and solar eclipses. During an eclipse, a particular universal energy and its influence on the mind are said to be temporarily withdrawn, creating more inner freedom and a clearer glimpse into the emptiness.

As seen earlier, Svara Yoga teaches that every event in the great external cycles of time is mirrored in the inner time-cycle of the breath. This brings us to a final method for using the knowledge of svara to transcend svara—and the universe—by discovering the timeless moment hidden within our own breathing.

If there is an outer equinox, an outer full and empty moon, and an outer eclipse, then these must also exist within us. By learning where the breath reaches in these special moments during our breathing, we can find a doorway into moments of timelessness in each and every breath. Each such moment is an opportunity to realize our true nature in a moment beyond time, in an "in-between" state leading to liberation.

The Four Sandhyās – Junctions of Breath and Day

Begin by identifying the four Sandhyās within your own breath. Sit comfortably and observe your breathing as it comes in and goes out, without trying to change it in any way.

Let your breath be natural. Do not make it longer or shorter; do not try to speed it up, slow it down, or make it deeper. Just allow it to happen and quietly track the movement of air from the heart out to the "end of twelve" (either just outside the nose or above the head), and notice what you feel.

Be aware of inhalation as it happens by itself: the expansion of the chest, the sensation of air flowing in through the nose, down the throat, and into the body.

Be aware of exhalation as it happens by itself: the air rising back up through the throat and leaving through the nose.

During this mediation, the breath may change in many ways, but over time you will usually notice that it begins to quiet down, becoming slower and more subtle.

If you continue, you may start to sense a slight pause at the end of inhalation, when the lungs are full and awareness rests in the chest, and another slight pause at the end of exhalation, when the lungs are empty and awareness is at the "end of the twelve".

With longer practice, you might also notice that sometimes the breath halts briefly in the middle of inhalation or in the middle of exhalation, around the back of the throat at the level of the uvula—though this is rarer and tends to arise only in deeper meditations.

These four special points are the Four Sandhyās of the breath.

1. The **Morning Sandhyā,** equivalent to sunrise, is the junction between inhalation and exhalation, when the lungs are completely full. It is the inner dawn in the heart, illuminating the Self beyond duality. From here the breath begins to exhale, and according to the tradition this activates the solar, warm piṅgalā nāḍī—one reason the outgoing breath tends to feel warm.
2. The **Mid-day Sandhyā,** corresponding to solar noon (Abhijit Muhurta), is the middle point of exhalation. This is the inner equinox, the madhya—the center point, equally distant from both inhalation and exhalation. "When night and day are equal, that is Viṣuvat, when inhalation and exhalation are equal, that is Suṣumṇā". At this moment the central channel, Suṣumṇā, is said to become active.
3. The **Evening Sandhyā,** equivalent to sunset, is the junction between exhalation and inhalation, at the end of the twelve (beyond the nose or above the crown of the head). This is a place

of peaceful repose, calmness, and a sense of inner emptiness. Here begins the inner night, the shift into the cooling, lunar iḍā nāḍī.

4. The **Mid-night Sandhyā** — Kālī's Hour — is the middle of inhalation, a moment of utter stillness in the outer world. At this point, the central channel is again said to become active.

All four Sandhyās are, in essence, moments of no breath (though the two "equinox" points of the breath only become truly breathless in very deep meditation). As the breath becomes breathless, we become timeless.

But why is this so? The only way to measure time is through change. If everything is completely still, there is nothing to mark the movement of time, and a direct experience of timelessness opens. In meditation, the body can become so still that, in a quiet environment, the only things that seem to "move" are breath and mind. If both of these come to rest, time stops, and even if this happens only for an instant, in that instant one tastes timeless eternity itself.

When the breath stops, the mind stops, because the two are intimately connected. Indian traditions teach that prāṇa is the cause of all motion in the world—wherever prāṇa goes, the mind goes, and when prāṇa ceases to move, everything that depended on it also becomes still.

When there is a moment of no breath, there is a moment of no movement of prāṇa. With no movement of prāṇa, there is no movement of mind—no mind means no inner events, no inner flow of time, and no way to sense whether time is passing or not; this is a glimpse of true timelessness.

The Junctions of breath with the monthly and yearly cycles

In the same way that we can map the four Sandhyās of the day onto the breath, we can also project other cycles of time into it, beginning with the monthly lunar cycle. The auspicious moment of the full moon, Pūrṇimā, is located at the end of exhalation, while the new moon, Amāvasyā, is found at the end of inhalation.

Similarly, the yearly solstices and equinoxes can be traced within the breath. The Winter Solstice is in the heart, when the breath comes to rest at the end of exhalation in the center of the chest, just before inhalation begins and the lungs are completely empty. The Summar Solstice is at the "end of the twelve", where exhalation ends and inhalation has not yet started, when the lungs are full. The Spring Equinox happens in the middle of inhalation, as the air reaches the uvula, and the Autumn Equinox occurs at the same place in the middle of exhalation.

These points are states of equilibrium between inhalation and exhalation, between the influence of prāṇa and apāna. They correspond to samāna vāyu and to the flow inside the Suṣumṇā. Therefore, in addition to the ordinary cycle of svara moving from left (iḍā, apāna) to right (piṅgalā, prāṇa), whenever the breath flows naturally through the Suṣumṇā—felt as the breath moving equally through both nostrils—it is said that we are in an inner "equinox moment".

"At the palate the breath changes direction; yogins focus there, for it is the equinox within". This is "the middle within the flow". It is also the location of khecarī mudrā (placing the tongue into the nasal cavity behind the uvula), a practice that can itself generate the timeless moment.

When we enter the space of this inner equinox and remain there, the movement in the Suṣumṇā—which is normally of the nature of samāna vāyu—turns into the rising udāna vāyu that lifts consciousness into higher states. Once the timeless moment is recognized, this movement resolves into the unmoving, all-pervasive vyāna vāyu, which is itself beyond time.

The *Śāradā-tilaka-Tantra* says: "By making use of the equinox (*Viṣuva-yoga*), one joins the soul to the eternal abode. He who attains the yoga of the equinox is freed from bondage".

Finally, there are moments known as internal eclipses. In the Indian tradition, an eclipse occurs when one celestial body "consumes" another; for Abhinavaputa, the author of the Tantaloka, the internal eclipse is each moment when one current entirely absorbs the other.

"A solar eclipse occurs when the lunar orb enters the solar orb; Rahu, the son of Siṁhikā, drinks the honey that flows from the moon".

The solar eclipse happens when the exhalation (the sun-current) is briefly absorbed into Suṣumṇā just before the next inhalation begins, and the lunar eclipse happens each time the inhalation (the moon-current) is absorbed into Suṣumṇā at the end of inhalation. These are the same inner locations and moments as the solstices, seen from another angle and emphasizing a different aspect.

Here the sun (exhalation) represents outward cognition, the moon (inhalation) represents inner subjectivity, and Rāhu—the eclipse node, the gap between them—represents the ego. The inner eclipse is the moment when all three are superimposed on one another, symbolizing the fusion of subject, object and knowing that characterizes Samadhi.

All these teachings point to one sacred insight: in every breath there are four potential moments of timelessness. By gently focusing on these locations and "catching" the instant when the breath touches them, it becomes possible to slip into the timeless moment; going beyond time, one becomes free and may experience the liberating eternity. The simplest way to explore this is with the meditation that opened this chapter: quietly observing the breath and giving extra attention to one, several, or all of these points along its path, until, in one of them, time simply stops.

Going beyond time in the Kalottara tantra

The *Kalottara Tantra* is an early (possibly 7th-century) scripture that describes liberation as entry into a timeless mode of existence. Together with the *Niśvāsa corpus*, it may be among the oldest sources teaching what later traditions call Svara and Kālacakra. Since this text has never been translated before, I will present some key verses along with brief explanations.

While most other tantras describe the highest state of consciousness in terms of universality or complete emptiness (a perspective of space), or as identification with universal consciousness (a perspective of knowing or being), the Kalottara is unique in that it portrays the highest consciousness primarily from the perspective of time. It teaches that the process of purification that leads to enlightenment is itself driven by time: "The blazing flame of time burns all darkness" (Kalottara in 100 verses).

It also insists that without knowledge of the inner cycles of time, liberation is impossible: "Without knowing subtle time, there is no siddhi or liberation" (Kalottara 150, 2.25).

Like other tantras, the Kalottara outlines various methods and rituals including: mantra, visualization, and initiation as gateways into the timeless state. At its heart, however, lies a technique that is characteristic of almost all tantras itself an elaboration of an older Upanishadic method of ascending a ladder of experiences from gross to subtle, from outer to inner. These experiences are usually mapped along the spine, with coarser experiences associated with the lower parts of the body and subtler ones with the upper body and beyond. The same ascent is also projected onto the breath, which travels from the heart (or lower) to the "end of the twelve" above the head.

This movement of consciousness is described as passing through the different elements that make up our reality: from the earth, to water, to fire, to air, to space, to mind, and beyond. Each element (tattva) is linked with a distinct level of consciousness. Beyond the mind and its senses, awareness enters a more fundamental sense of pure being, and finally moves past even that into experiences of universal consciousness. These progressively subtler states are often symbolized as ascending to the levels of various deities such as Brahmā, Viṣṇu, and Śiva.

> "By exhalation the yogin casts upward the prāṇa, and through mastery lifts the heart-lotus, establishing it in the upward stream.
>
> The exhaled prāṇa ascends upward, piercing the knot in a moment, and having pierced the skull-gate, the soul rises upward".
>
> (Kalottara 350, 10.49-50)

Different tantric lineages list these divinities and what they symbolize in different orders. The Kalottara, the "beyond time" tantra, is dedicated to Śiva as the very element of time, the creator and transcender of time: "Maheśvara manifests as time itself, taking the universal form" (Kalottara 150, 2.16). "Salutations to you, knower and transcender of time. Salutations to you, Lord of time, the one who sets all cycles of time in motion" (Kalottara 150 1.1). From this perspective, the highest reality is described as that which lies beyond Śiva—that is, beyond time and causality.

The Kalottara is also the earliest extant text to clearly teach the method for condensing internal time in order to speed up evolution: "Sixty years are said to be one full day and night for yogis (one breath)" Kalottara 150, 2.3), and "That day and night which I declared to you, is known as a year in the Tantra named 'Kāla'" (Kalottara 150, 2.8).

In addition, the Kalottara is among the first to teach that balancing the flow of the left and right nāḍīs and drawing the prāṇa into the central channel creates an inner equinox. This inner equinox is presented as the doorway into the liberating, timeless moment:

> "When the Self enters the central channel, the wise know that to be the inner equinox" (Kalottara 100).
>
> "In the middle lies the equinox (viṣuvam), flowing equally through both channels (nostrils)" (Kalottara 700, 10.40).
>
> "All actions should be undertaken through inner time. For the liberation-seeker, the offering (yajana) in viṣuva is especially praised" (Kalotarra 150 2.22).
>
> "By the equinox-union (viṣuva-yoga) one should be established in the timeless state. Having attained the viṣuva-yoga, who would not be freed from bondage?" (Kalottara 200, 5.15)

And this process is said to be internally tied to the natural rhythm of alternation between the nostrils.

> "By the alternation of left and right flows, in half-yāma cycles (24 minutes), The Rudra-tattva is first said to arise through Piṅgalā".

These may be the oldest surviving teachings on Svara Yoga and its relationship to the timeless moment.

Timelessness in the Vedas and Upanishads

Though the teachings of the Kalottara, and even more so Abhinavagupta's *Tantraloka*, are among the clearest when it comes to defining the universal state of consciousness as going beyond time, the oldest roots of this insight appear already in the *Ṛgveda*. In *the Nāsadīya Sūkta* (Ṛgveda 10.129), there is a description of a state before creation in which time has not yet arisen: "Death was not then, nor was there immortality. There was no sign of night, nor of day".

A little later, the *Kaṭha Upaniṣad* presented a dialogue between the boy Naciketas and Yama, the Lord of Death, in which Naciketasa sks about ultimate reality and Yama replies by describing the timeless nature of the Absolute. Yama teaches that the Puruṣa (Self or soul) is "the Lord of the past and the future", who is "the same today and tomorrow", and that "The intelligent Self is not born, nor does It die... It is unborn, eternal, everlasting, ancient..." All of this points to a state of eternal presence that is not bound by the linear progression of time.

Similarly, the *Śvetāśvatara Upaniṣad* (6.6 & 6.5) refers to the Supreme Being as the one who transcends time, going beyond the three dimensions of time—past, present, and future.

The Timeless Eternal "Block Universe"

To close this chapter, it helps to jump from some of the oldest teachings on "timelessness" to some of the most modern.

In modern physics, space and time are not two separate things; together they form a single four-dimensional structure called spacetime. Instead of picturing the universe as three dimensions of space in which objects move while time flows past, spacetime treats time as another dimension, similar to the three dimensions of space.

Every event—every place, every moment—is a point in this four-dimensional "block". In this view, nothing "flows" through time and nothing truly comes and goes. Rather, the entire past, present, and future of the universe already exists together as a complete, static structure.

From our human perspective, it feels as if time moves forward because we experience the block one "slice" at a time. But in the spacetime model itself, past, present, and future are all equally real, and the universe appears as a timeless, four-dimensional whole.

In essence, modern physics suggests that the universe may be fundamentally timeless, and that our experience of time is emergent or perspectival—a feature of how we perceive reality, not a basic property of reality itself.

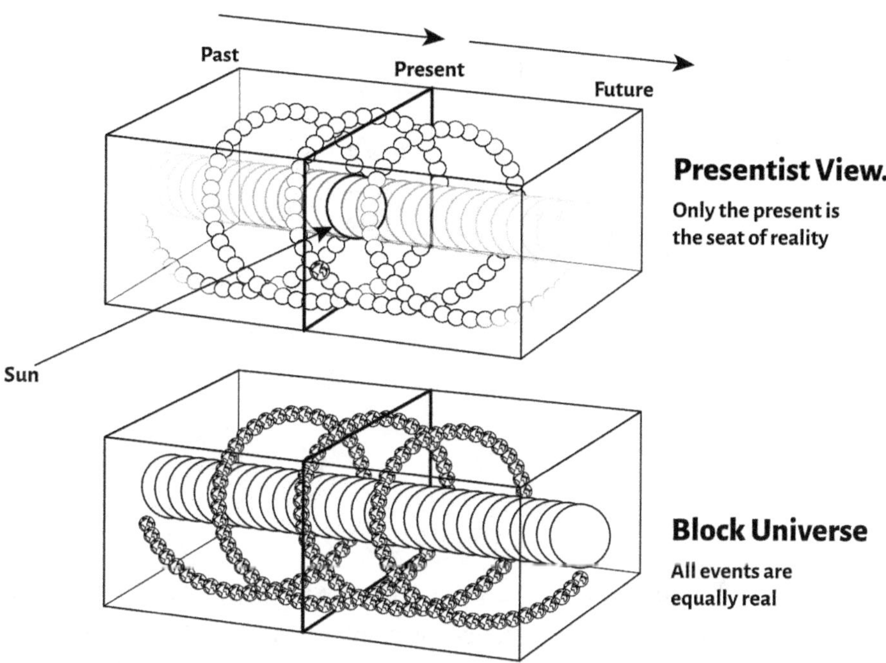
Past
Present
Future
Presentist View.
Only the present is the seat of reality
Sun
Block Universe
All events are equally real

Chapter 31
Kālī, The Goddess Who is Time and Devours Time

In this final chapter I want to share with you what may both be the most approachable and the most radical way of working with Time in the tantric Indian tradition: with time not as a "what", but a "whom".

The Tantric traditions teach that the entire universe is born out of consciousness, and that everything is, in fact conscious. We are conscious; animals and plants are conscious; rocks (to a degree), planets, the sun, the galaxy, even space are conscious—and time itself is conscious.

If time were conscious, what would his?! her?! it's?! awareness be like? It would certainly be detached, because he, she, they would know with absolute clarity that everything passes; from our side, it might appear cruel, destroying everything we cling to, yet in truth it would have to be profoundly compassionate. Because Time would be the father or mother of everything that happens, since nothing can "happen" without time. In the Indian tradition, this living, consciousness has been given the name Kālī—a name that simultaneously means "the dark one" and "Time".

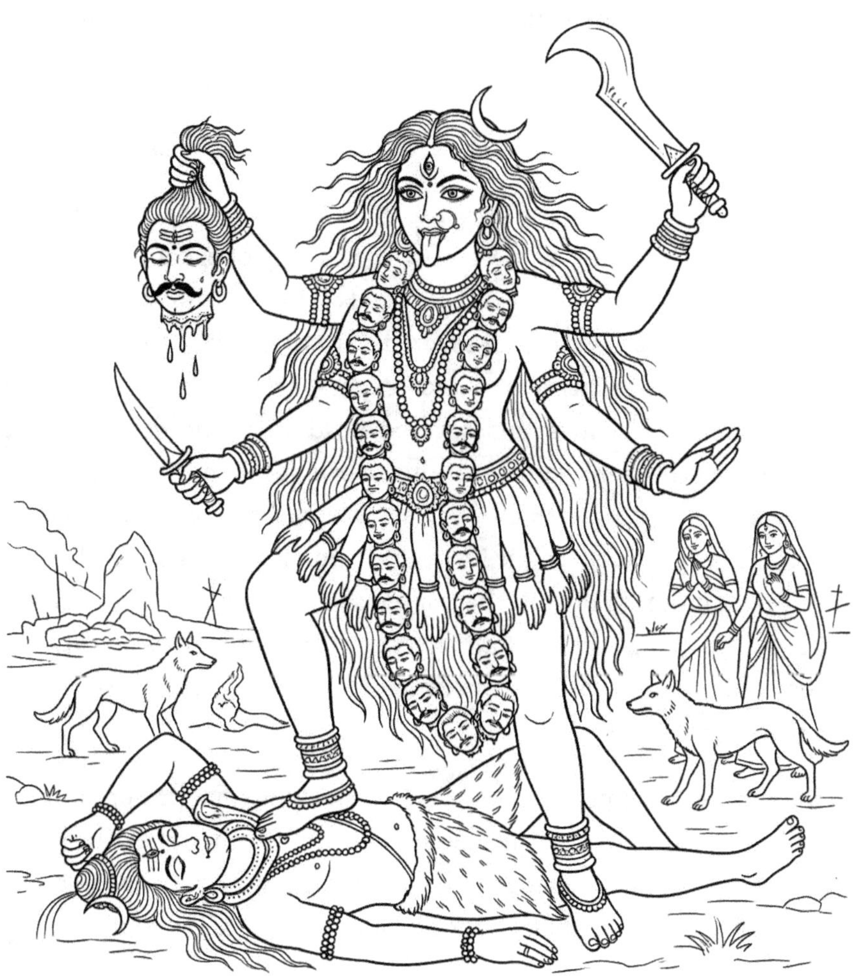

Who is Kālī?

Kālī is usually depicted standing naked in the middle of a cremation ground, with one foot placed on the motionless body of Śiva. This highlights her independence and supremacy in Śākta theology, and her power as the animating force behind Śiva —for without her feminine power (codified in the letter ī), Śiva is nothing but a śava, a corpse.

The cremation ground further emphasizes her domain: the place where all forms end, and Kālī as the end of time itself, where all existence dissolves. Her blackness is not evil, but the void at the end of time into which everything returns, and her nakedness reflects unvarnished reality, free from social covering. Her wild, unbound hair signals autonomy and a refusal to be domesticated by conventional order.

The rest of her iconography expands the same message. She wears a garland of severed heads, representing the cutting of ego and the letters of speech, indicating that she both ends illusion and generates all expression. She wears a girdle of severed arms, symbolizing mastery over action (karma), while her four hands express her dual nature: the left hands holding the cleaver and severed head show the destruction of ignorance, and the right hands granting fearlessness and boons show her protective, liberating side. Kālī's protruding tongue—whether interpreted as shock or as an insatiable appetite for ego-dissolution—points to her power to devour the limited self. Surrounded by jackals and spirits, beings of thresholds, Kālī appears as the force that rules the in-between and reveals that freedom comes not from avoiding darkness but from seeing through it.

Despite her fearful appearance, more than most Indian representations of the divine, it is Kālī who is considered the loving mother of all the beings in the universe. Like a mother, she is the one who watches over her children as they grow up, by making time move and allowing them to develop.

In many depictions, Kālī is independent and alone; in this sense she is both time—past, present, and future—and that which is beyond time. In other depictions she has a male consort known as Mahākāla; there, he is time itself, and she, MahaKālī, is the one who devours time, the eternal, timeless being at the end of time.

> "Thou art the Night of Time (Kālarātri); Thou art Peace; verily Thou art the supreme Prakṛti".
>
> - Kālikā Purāṇa Chapter 8 verse 23

What Kālī brings to our lives

To work with the spiritual force of Kālī is to work with time itself. This means not being limited by time, but being aided by time. Time is a precious commodity. We need time in order to evolve, yet for most of us time seems to run out far too fast.

A common teaching in the Indian tradition is that reaching enlightenment requires multiple lifetimes and countless years. Kriyā Yoga is said to have been designed to speed up this process, but even Kriyā Yoga is still fighting against the force of time. To work with Kālī—to worship Kālī—means to make friends with time, to have time on your side.

Kālī is considered a catalyst of transformation, compressing what might have been a slow evolution into an intense burst of growth. The friendship of time will bring us what we need for our evolution, even when it is painful to receive. This is why her iconography is so terrible: to work with her is to experience, in one lifetime, the kinds of lessons we might otherwise face over many lifetimes—a sped up evolution.

The psychologist Erik Erickson famously divided life into stages of development—a very Kālī-like endeavor. He taught that the final stage, "Integrity versus Despair", centers on how a person reflects on their life in their last years: whether they arrive at "integrity"—a sense of fulfillment and wholeness from a life well lived—or fall into "despair", marked by regret and bitterness over an unfulfilled, meaningless life.

Kālī makes sure that our lives are filled with meaningful moments to grow from. A devotee of Kālī may feel the sharp pains of growth, but is spared the heavier melancholy of stagnation.

Ramakrishna is a famous example of this accelerated evolution. He practiced the disciplines of dozens of paths—Tantra, Vaiṣṇavism, Islam, Christianity, and more—within just a few years, achieving the goal of each path in days what others are said to require lifetimes to realize. This supernatural speed is attributed to the grace of the Divine Mother Kālī, who "pushed" him through these realizations, compressing the spiritual history of humanity into a single biography. But this hastened evolution also came at a cost: toward the end of his life Ramakrishna developed throat cancer, and he continued to teach though that his suffering was part of the Mother's "play".

The 18th-century Bengali poet Ramprasad Sen offers perhaps the most poignant "insider" view of the suffering inherent in Kālī worship. His songs (*Rāmprasādi*) are not polite hymns; they are complaints, lawsuits, and cries of anguish addressed directly to the Mother. He accuses her of being heartless: "I'm sick of living, Mother, sick. Life and money have all run out... You make and break. You've broken me in this life". He writes of the "pitiless funerals of the poor" and the raw fear of death, giving voice to the way Kālī's love can feel from inside a life she is relentlessly transforming.

Yet within Ramprasad's complaint lies a clear recognition of the mechanism at work. In one of his most famous songs, he uses the image of a kite flying in the sky: the Mother holds the string and plays with the kite, making it swoop and dive. The string is coated with manja, a paste made of ground glass. This glass represents the suffering and difficulties of the world, but its purpose is not to torture the kite; it is to make the string sharp enough to cut itself. When the string cuts, the kite is free. Ramprasad sings: "Out of a hundred thousand kites, at best but one or two break free; And thou dost laugh and clap Thy hands, O Mother, watching them!"

Across the traditions there is a recurring warning: to invoke Kālī is to invite the experience of death while still alive. If one is not "ready"—if the vessel is not baked strong enough—the influx of this energy can lead to madness or physical destruction. The "burning of karma" brings great clarity, but if one burns up the entire karmic stock too quickly, the body may not be able to withstand it.

Working with her, however, Kālī not only accelerates of one's evolution through the speeding up of inner time, but she also becomes a doorway into the timeless moment itself. The aim of yogic states is union with the object of meditation. To become united with Kālī is to be united with the timeless moment itself, so that any meditation on Kālī, if performed properly, becomes an experience of the liberating, timeless moment.

How to bring Kālī's influence into your life

Similar to the work with other goddesses, there are three main ways to bring Kālī's presence into our lives and to access the timeless through her.

1. Bhakti

The simplest and most direct way to worship Kālī, is through bhakti—the raw and intimate devotion that places one's whole heart at the Mother's feet. The bhakta seeks to connect with the object of devotion on a personal level; it is an intimate relationship with the divine. In bhakti, one may relate to Kālī either as one's child, as one's lover, but most naturally and powerfully as one's own mother.

What does a bhakta do? They think about their beloved, praise them, seek them, and worship them.

Ramprasad sang to Kālī while working in the fields or sitting before his household shrine, offering nothing more than simple flowers, a bit of incense, and the whole of his longing—often calling her "Ma" and speaking to her as naturally as to a living mother.

Ramakrishna, serving as priest of the Dakshineswar Kālī temple, would sometimes abandon formal ritual altogether, simply weeping, call her name, or singing Ramprasad's songs until he lost outer consciousness and was engulfed in visions of his beloved.

In bhakti, love for the deity is gradually cultivated. Sometimes this takes a self-negating form, in which the beloved becomes everything that exists and "you" simply seem to disappear—like a parent whose whole world becomes their child, or a small child who feels the mother is the entire universe. Sometimes it appears as the longing of lovers who wish so deeply to unite that they embrace and try to become one body in sexual ecstasy.

What happens when one becomes one with Kālī? Quite simply, one becomes one with the timeless moment; through love directed towards this form, this personification, one may attain the transcendence of svara.

2. Pūjā & sādhana

In December of 2011, at the height of a lunar eclipse in a sacred cremation ground in eastern Bihar, among various sādhus and candle-lit human skulls, I received my full initiation into Kālī's sādhana—a practice that has shaped me ever since.

One of the main ways of working with Kālī is through what is known as pūjā and sādhana. Pūjā means ritual worship. It can include working with her yantra, the spiritual diagram that embodies her form, or with her rūpa, her iconographic image. Such practice may involve many symbolical acts of offering, the performance of fire rituals, and sacred pilgrimages. This outer ritual is combined with daily practice of one of her secret mantras; together they invite her living presence into one's life.

3. Mantra

Perhaps the most profound of all the practices of working with Kālī is the use of her mantra. In the Indian tradition, the mantra is considered to be the very body of the deity, so to repeat her mantra is to allow Kālī herself to be expressed through your being.

Mantra sādhana is usually done seated on a special meditation cloth, an āsan, while repeating her mantra—either in a whisper or in absolute silence. The practice may involve repeating the mantra hundreds of thousands of times.

With each repetition, it's as if a little more of her energy is imbibed into our being. The more the sādhana is done, the more her presence accumulates in our lives, and the more our lives begin to be shaped by her will. The practice can continue until one becomes so completely suffused with her that life itself becomes a playground through which she guides and moves.

To work with most mantras, however, one must receive proper initiation; without it, the mantra may not work or could even be harmful. This is why most of Kālī's mantras remain secret.

Still, there are some mantras of Kālī that are openly known, and one such mantra is:

"*Om Krīm Kālikāyai Namaḥ*"

This mantra can be repeated by anyone who wishes to invite her presence more fully into their life. It is traditionally recommended to recite it only when you feel clean both physically and emotionally, after taking a bath. For women, it is advised not to use this mantra during menstruation—not because menstruation is impure, but because during this time the woman is considered to be suffused with a particular form of another divine goddess known as Mātangi, and during this time one can only work with that specific form. Though I write this mantra here, it is important to keep in mind the warnings offered by her devotees.

The Kalikrama's teachings on Kālī within us

The final, and perhaps most esoteric, way of working with Kālī, unique to her, appears in the Kalikrama ("sequence of Kālī") tradition, where Kālīis said to manifest in our very act of cognition.

According to the Kālī-krama, the entire cycle of creation, maintenance, and destruction of the universe can be seen in every single act of knowing. For what is cognition, if not the creation of an inner representation of the world within the emptiness of the mind, followed by its dissolution back into the silence beyond thought?

The Kalikrama divides this act of cognition into twelve steps, each personified as a different Kālī; together, the Twelve Kālīs embody the whole cycle of time, consciousness, and cosmic processes. Presiding over them all is Kāla Saṃkarṣiṇī, the Kālī who is beyond time and devours time. In the body, she is said to dwell at the midpoint behind the palate, halfway along the flow of the breath—so the entire process can also be mapped onto the svara of inhaling and exhaling.

Although this teaching is traditionally considered "secret", it was nontheless expounded by tantric masters like Abhinavagupta in works such as his *Tantrāloka* and the *Krama-stotra.*

The process of perception begins with the creation of the universe with Śṛṣṭi Kāli, the Kālīof Emanation—the first surge of pure awareness eager to manifest objectivity. Next comes Rakta Kāli, the *Kāli* of Persistence, where consciousness turns outward in delight to experience the universe with joy. When she grows weary of this outwardness, Stiti-nāśa Kālī, the Kālī of the Destruction of Persistence, appears. The fourth, Yama Kālī -the Kālī of Restriction—is the transitional state between creation and dissolution, the moment when doubt about the solid reality of the external world arises. Then Saṃhāra Kālī, the fifth Kālī, emerges, withdrawing the senses and the external world back into herself so that the universe is experienced within. The sixth is Mṛtyu Kālī ,Kālī of Death, when even individuality dissolves into pure perception. After this, Rudra Kālī appears as a deeper layer of doubt; this doubt allows the ego to reappear temporarily with Mātṛka Kālī , the Kālī of the Sun, who makes us believe "we" are the doer—until it is recognized that this "we" does not exist, and that it is truly Kālī who perceives and acts through us. The ninth is Paramārka Kālī, the Kālī of the Supreme Sun, who unites the personal "I" with the universal "I", like a sun-ray returning to its source. Kālāgni Rudra Kālī, the Kālī of the Fire of Time, stabilizes the presence of Śiva in action—acting as the divine agent while burning away time in the form of karma. Next Mahākāla Kālī, the Kālī of Great Time, manifests when all karmas have been exhausted and the yogin moves from eternal time rather than sequential time. Finally comes Mahābhairava Ghora Caṇḍā Kālī, the Kali of the Great Terrible Bhairava, the final form in this sequence. She represents the ultimate, most intense manifestation of Kālī's power—in which all subjects, objects, and means of knowledge dissolve into pure consciousness where only a single, undivided awareness remains. With this, Śakti merges back into Śiva, ending a cycle.

The Krama as Cognitive Yoga

The Krama system of Mother Kālī teaches that we are bound because we do not know the nature of time. Liberation arises from perceiving the birth, duration, and dissolution of every moment, which means total and continuous presence.

Thus, a yogi who knows the nature of birth, persistence, and reabsorption is liberated, while those who do not know it are pervaded solely by bondage. Buddhism describes this as the realization of transitoriness—that nothing is permanent—while the Kalikrama seems the same event and names it the play and pulsation of Kālī.

According to these teachings, the process of perception can be merged with the breath: inhalation equated to withdrawal (saṃhāra), exhalation with manifestation (sṛṣṭi), and the holding of the air with the ineffable (anākhyā).

In Krama practice, the practitioner directs awareness inward even as perception flows outward. This inward gaze, comparable to the Tibetan Mahāmudrā, yields direct perception of the phases of consciousness—the twelve moments of arising and dissolution.

To observe our perception is to watch the fastest events that unfold in our lives, since anything shorter than perception itself cannot be perceived. The smallest units of time are the closest to the timeless moment, because timelessness means no passing of time, and the passing of a very short moment is closer to the non-passing than a longer one—just as the number 1 is closer to 0 than the number 5.

Thus by focusing on perception, the yogi comes closest to the timeless moment itself, which is the "place" from which perception is observed (for to see time, one much look from beyond time). Being so close to the timeless moment makes it easier to recognize it, and therefore easier for the yogi to awaken to their own timeless essence.

The Svara Yoga Epilogue: Integrating Svara Yoga for Your Own Evolution

Congratulations to making it to the end of this book. Thank you for joining me on this journey and staying with it all the way to this point. In this final chapter, the aim is to revisit what we have explored together and to offer some new guidance on how to adapt these teachings to your own life and practice.

The Foundation: Humanity and Natural Cycles

We began by unraveling the profound connection between humanity and the cyclical patterns of nature. From the shifting seasons to the dance of celestial bodies, we saw how these rhythms have woven themselves into our collective consciousness through myths and stories.

We then discovered an ancient Indian science that helps us align our actions with these cycles as they manifest both in the body and in the universe, helping us to minimize resistance and maximize success: the science of Svara Yoga.

We learned that the practice of Svara Yoga harnesses the power of the breath in a way distinct from prāṇāyāma or simple breath-awareness meditation, focusing on analyzing the breath to discern the inner rhythms of the body. The key element being the flow of the air as it passes through the right or left nostril, which termed svara, gives its name to the system.

We also learned that this is a scientifically recognized pattern called the nasal cycle, and that understanding its connection to the two brain hemispheres and the autonomic nervous system helps to illuminate the workings of Svara Yoga.

From there, we turned to the traditional explanation of how this cycle affects the being through the subtle physiology of the yogic body, exploring nāḍīs, chakras, and kośas. We studied the three primary nāḍīs—Iḍā, Piṅgalā, and Suṣumnā—their relationship to the three guṇas (sattva, rajas, and tamas), and their resonance with the yin-yang division of chi.

Practical Applications: Aligning Actions with Svara

After understanding the theoretical basis, we turned to the main practical aspect of Svara Yoga: We first learned how to identify the svara, and then continued with the actions recommended to be done or avoided during each svara, learning how to tap into the lunar, solar, and śūnya svara for optimal results.

We also saw that the traditional list of guidelines is relatively minimal and at times confusing, so we explored the scientific foundations of Svara Yoga, connecting it to the sympathetic and parasympathetic nervous systems and the differing functions of the left and right brain hemispheres. This exploration gave us a broader understanding of what Svara Yoga is really about and empowered us to begin forming our own intuitive guidelines regarding what is best done on the left svara and what is best done on the right.

After learning the basics of what is recommended in each svara, we examined the effects of overactivation in either system and explored techniques for restoring equilibrium to the autonomic nervous system. We studied methods for shifting the breath from one nostril to the other, giving us powerful tools to influence the direction of our lives.

We also gained practical insight into ways of aligning our actions with the flow of svara throughout the day, from the moment of waking to the moment of falling asleep, so that the entire daily routine can be optimized for maximum effectiveness.

Adding Complexity: Elements and Cosmic Influences

After studying the basics of breath, we began to add more layers to understand its complexities. We explored the meeting point between cosmic energies and everyday life, seeing how each day of the week resonates with a specific planetary influence. This understanding, combined with Svara Yoga, offers a powerful matrix for aligning your actions so that external astrological forces and your internal svara rhythm can move in harmony.

The chapter on recognizing breath length shed light on the subtle messages encoded in the duration of each inhale and exhale, and how these rhythms quietly impact your physical, mental, and emotional state.

We then learned a profound prāṇāyāma with a one-four-two-one ratio, a pattern that attunes us with the sacred flow of prāṇa and opens a gateway to expand vitality and awareness. The guided haṃsa meditation introduced an ancient, universal way of breathing that bridges individual and universal consciousness, offering a direct pathway to inner peace and realization.

We turned to the five elements, pañcatattva, and uncovered some of the ancient wisdom behind these foundational forces of existence. In the chapter on the elemental cycle within the breath, we saw how the ongoing dance of earth, water, fire, air, and ether continually colors each breath and participates in shaping our karmic journey.

We reviewed practical tools for recognizing which tattva is predominant at a given moment, so our self-awareness can become more precise and our choices more aligned with these subtle cycles. One tool introduced was to use the condensation patterns on a mirror as a simple, grounded means to observe the active tattva in your svara.

We also learned Śāṇmukī mudrā, a powerful technique for sensing which tattva is alive in the inner space of your being.

Finally, we explored how actions bear different results depending on which element is present, offering concrete insight into how to time and shape your efforts in daily life—like learning to coordinate your actions with the dominant nostril or breath flow.

We also learned how to practice Trāṭaka, or steady gazing, on the elemental symbols, and how this simple, focused act can deepen your understanding of the elements themselves.

Additional Cycles from Eastern Traditions

Having completed the exploration of elemental flow, we then opened the door to several other cycles from Eastern traditions. We began with the Ayurvedic clock and its dynamic interplay of the three doṣas, noticing how their rhythms influence daily energy shifts and enrich our understanding of the svaras and tattvas.

The Chinese Chi clock added another layer, mapping the flow of the vital life force through specific organs and showing how this circulation influences physical, mental, and emotional states through the lens of the Chinese tradition.

We then turned to the astrological planetary hours, or horas, as preserved from ancient Babylon sources. This system expanded the earlier study of days and their corresponding elements by revealing which planetary influence is active during hour, refining the way we sense and track subtle energetic tides throughout the day.

Specialized applications: Birth, Death, and Divination

From there, we touched on Svara Śāstra's insight into pregnancy, while also recognizing the patrilineal worldview embedded in these traditional texts. Within that frame, we considered their teachings on conception and on determining the sex of a child, hopefully approaching them with both curiosity and discernment.

The exploration continued from birth to death, as we studied the ancient methods—rooted in Tibetan Tantra—for contemplating and predicting the moment of one's passing, offering a unique perspective into how these traditions relate to life's ultimate transition.

Finally, we tasted a drop of the mystical realm of Svara Yoga, through its applications in divination, seeing how breath and elemental wisdom can inform practices like astrology and tarot, and offering a glimpse into how much more we can learn from the science of Svara Yoga beyond this introductory journey.

The Svara Transcended

At the end of this journey, Svara Yoga reveals its deepest promise: not only harmony with the rhythms of nature, but the discovery of the freedom that shines beyond them. Through the purification of the Kalachakra, the accelerated evolution of Kriya, the stillness of the Sandhyas, and the fierce grace of Kali, the breath emerged as the final threshold between the bound and the liberated. By mastering the inner zodiac and attuning to the timeless pauses between inhalation and exhalation, we learned that the yogi can transform time itself into a vehicle of awakening, stepping out of the wheel of karma into the eternal, unconditioned now, where breather, breath, and time dissolve into absolute freedom.

The Approach of This Book

In shaping this book, I tried to make this cycle of teachings as complete, yet as clear and succinct, as possible. I tried to present the tradition in a way that is contemporary and scientific, while still honoring the authenticity and depth of the original sources.

Having reviewed this journey, I'd like to offer a more modern lens on how you might apply these teachings personally, moving from the book knowledge that Svara Yoga offers us into lived, embodied wisdom.

Beyond One-Size-Fits-All Approaches

Svara Yoga, as shared here, shows how external astrological cycles—the rising and falling of the sun, the phases of the moon, and the movement of the planets—affect our inner cycles, which in turn influence how we think, feel, and act.

Yet a central limitation appears: these teachings largely overlook individual constitution.

When Svara Yoga is understood as a balance between the sympathetic and parasympathetic nervous systems, and between the right and left brain hemispheres, a doorway opens to adapt the practices of this knowledge to different nervous system types and psychological profiles.

If someone already lives with a hyperactivated sympathetic system, how should they apply the knowledge of Svara Yoga? Should they practice in the same way as everyone else, or are intelligent adaptations needed? This question is offered deliberately as an open invitation for inquiry, experimentation, and future exploration, rather than something with a fixed answer.

Understanding Individual Differences

We are each different, shaped not only by the events of our lives but also by how those events imprinted on our nervous system. On top of that, our unique genetic makeup adds another layer of distinction, creating deeply personal patterns of response and perception.

Western psychologies suggest that genetic makeup—together with what happens during pregnancy in utero—can create three broad newborn temperaments: easy-going, slow-to-warm, and active. These early patterns offer a helpful lens for understanding why different people may experience and respond to the same Svara in very different ways.

Temperament Type	Nervous System Balance	Characteristics
Easy-going	Balanced between sympathetic and parasympathetic	Generally adaptable and calm
Slow-to-warm	More parasympathetic	Cautious, need time to adjust
Active	More sympathetic	High energy, quick to react

We can map these three basic infant temperaments to an inborn balance between the parasympathetic and sympathetic nervous systems. The easy-going type reflects a more balanced state, slow-to-warm leans toward parasympathetic dominance, and the active type tends toward sympathetic dominance. Each of us starts life with a different nervous system tendency, which then evolves and is amplified by everything that happens to us over the years.

The Impact of Life Experience

When life brings repeated or intense trauma, our system, regardless of its baseline tends to become even more imbalanced, wither tilting toward parasympathetic freezing and shutdown, or toward sympathetic overdrive and chronic anxiety. With this in mind, the intention of this final chapter is to offer ways of adapting Svara Yoga to your specific history, life conditions, and personality, rather than assuming a single formula fits everyone.

Personalizing the Practice: A Practical Example

Classical Svara Yoga often teaches that when we want to be strong, assertive, and forceful, we should emphasize breathing through the right nostril. But I'd invite you to look more closely: if you already tend to be overly aggressive or confrontational, it may be more skillful for you to enter negotiation supported by a parasympathetic, lunar svara state instead.

In this way, the general guidelines remain useful, but when combined with honest self-knowledge and understanding—what comes easily, where there are blind spots or deficiencies—the entire system becomes truly adaptable and deeply personal.

Understanding Your Personal Baseline

I invite you to gather everything you already know about yourself and place it within a simple yet powerful question: Am I more parasympathetically activated, or more sympathetically activated?

You revisit the chapters on the nature of the Iḍā and Piṅgalā nāḍīs, along with the scientific foundations of Svara Yoga, and use either a more spiritual lens or a more scientific one—as long as you arrive at a clear understanding of what "more" means in your own case, relative to the following:

Lunar/Parasympathetic Qualities	Solar/Sympathetic Qualities
Lunar	Solar
Yin	Yang
Iḍā nāḍī activated	Right nostril
Left nostril	Piṅgalā nāḍī
Right brain	Left brain hemisphere
Parasympathetic	Sympathetic activated

Once you have a sense of your baseline—more sympathetic or more parasympathetic—the next step is to notice how this pattern appears in your life. Ask yourself honestly: What are you normally? How has this shaped the choices you make?

Retrospective Analysis

You can look back at various situations and gently inquire: if there had been less sympathetic activation, or less parasympathetic withdrawal, how might this situation have turned out differently?

Rather than following the black-and-white guidelines of the *Śiva Svarodaya*, simply begin to decide for yourself: if in a certain type of situation you clearly needed more sympathetic activation, then next time, consciously shift the breath to the right nostril before you step into it. On the contrary, if you recognize that more left-nostril, parasympathetic breathing would likely have brought a wiser outcome, then you can choose that instead.

Building Your Personal Map

It's important not to get stuck in regret or fantasy about the past. We cannot look back and say, "Oh, I should have done *that*". You cannot truly know what would have happened, but you can analyze, experiment a few times in similar conditions, and notice: "In this kind of situation, I function better when I'm more parasympathetic", or the opposite.

After a few times, this experiment-based learning reveals your own map, where growing self-knowledge naturally drives self-growth and allows Svara Yoga to be tailored to your own personal constitution.

Practical Application and Long-term Perspective

As a reminder, Svara Yoga speaks about changes in karma, and karmic changes can take a long time to manifest. These shifts move on a much longer timescale than immediate feedback. When you evaluate whether an action—or a particular svara choice—was successful, look not only at the short-term result but also what unfolds months or even years later. And that, of course, depends on the situation.

If the situation is something short-term, like a negotiation, you will usually sense within a week or two whether your approach—and your svara choice—was effective. But with long-term questions, such as buying a house, it may take decades to truly recognize if that was a beneficial decision. For decisions on that kind of long horizon, where you cannot really run experiments, I would recommend to follow the guidelines of the *Śiva Svarodaya* as they are. I believe there's no harm in that.

But for more immediate, repeatable situations—specific interactions where you can observe results over months or a year—you can actively experiment and refine your own map of when to emphasize parasympathetic or sympathetic activation, right or left brain, and evolve your own individual path that adapts Svara Yoga to your personal constitution.

Closing Meditation and Reflections

To close, I want to invite you to take one minute of meditation. Sit comfortably with your spine erect and observe your breath. Notice which nostril is more open and active, and, if possible, sense which element is present in the svara at this very moment.

With this awareness, gently meditate on how everything you have learned here might reshape your life. How might your days unfold if each action were as optimal as possible, if you continuously gave yourself the best conditions to succeed and to grow? Let your mind rest for a minute in the felt possibility of a future in which this knowledge it is fully lived.

Thank you again for walking with me on this journey and for your willingness to look so closely at breath, karma, and consciousness. May these teachings support your growth, revealing something new about both the vast universe and your own deepest nature.

Oṃ Śānti, Śānti, Śānti.

Bibliography

Abhinavagupta. *Tantrāloka: The Light on and of the Tantras - Volume Six (Chapters Nine and Ten).* With the commentary *Viveka* by Jayaratha. Translated and edited by Mark S. G. Dyczkowski. Varanasi: Indological Resources, 2012.

Bhavanani, Ananda Balayogi. 'Swarodaya Vigjnan: A Scientific Study of the Nasal Cycle.' Yoga Mimamsa 39 (2007): 32–38.

Dorje, Gyurme, trans. *The Tibetan Book of the Dead.* Edited by Graham Coleman and Thupten Jinpa. New York: Penguin Classics, 2007.

Goodall, Dominic, ed. *Niśvāsatattvasaṃhitā: The Earliest Surviving Śaiva Tantra.* Pondicherry: Institut Français de Pondichéry, 2015.

Hand, Robert. *Night & Day: Planetary Sect in Classical Astrology.* Reston, VA: ARHAT Publications, 1995.

Jella, Susan A., and David S. Shannahoff-Khalsa. "The effects of unilateral forced nostril breathing on cognitive performance." *International Journal of Neuroscience* 73, no. 1-2 (1993): 61-68.

Johari, Harish. *Breath, mind, and consciousness.* Inner Traditions/Bear & Co, 1989.

Kaivalyadhama Editorial board. *Śiva Svarodaya.* Critical Edition. Lonavala: Kaivalyadhama, 2015.

Kannan, S., trans. *Svara Cintāmaṇi*: Divination by Breath. Madras: Kannan Publications, 1967.

Kshirsagar, Suhas, and Michelle D. Seaton. *Change Your Schedule, Change Your Life: How to Harness the Power of Clock Genes to Lose Weight, Optimize Your Workout, and Finally Get a Good Night's Sleep*. New York: Harper Wave, 2018.

Muktibodhananda, Swami. *Swara Yoga: The Tantric Science of Brain Breathing*. Munger: Bihar School of Yoga, 1984.

Prasad, Rama. Nature's finer forces; the science of breath and the philosophy of the tattvas. London: Theosophical Publishing Society, 1894

Sarajit Poddar, *The Principles of Svara Shastra: A Journey into the World of Vedic Astrology*, In Search of Jyotish 25 (Chennai: Notion Press, 2023).

Śāstrī, Biswanarayan, trans. *Kalika Purana, 3 vols., text with translation and notes in English versewise by Biswanarayan Shastri*. Delhi: Nag Publishers, 1994.

Shannahoff-Khalsa, David S., and Brian Kennedy. "The effects of unilateral forced nostril breathing on the heart." International Journal of Neuroscience 73, no. 1-2 (1993): 47-60.

Shannahoff-Khalsa, David S., Michael R. Boyle, and Marcia E. Buebel. "The effects of unilateral forced nostril breathing on cognition." *International Journal of Neuroscience* 57, no. 3-4 (1991): 239-249.

Shannahoff-Khalsa, David. "The ultradian rhythm of alternating cerebral hemispheric activity." *International journal of neuroscience* 70, no. 3-4 (1993): 285-298.

Sivananda, Swami. *The Science of Pranayama*. 11th ed. Rishikesh: Divine Life Society, 1971.

Sivananda, Swami. *Svara Yoga*. 4th ed. Shivanandanagar, India: The Divine Life Society, 2011.

Ursinus, Lothar. The Body Clock in Traditional Chinese Medicine. Rochester, VT: Inner Traditions, 2020.

Vagbhata. *Vagbhata's Astanga Hrdayam: Text, English Translation, Notes, Appendix and Indices.* Translated by K.R. Srikantha Murthy. 3 vols. Varanasi: Krishnadas Academy, 2000.

Weiss, Tomer. "*Kālottara Tantra*." Unpublished manuscript. Retrieved from Muktabodha Indological Research Institute, 2025.

Weiss, Tomer. "Svacchanda Tantra." Unpublished manuscript. Retrieved from Muktabodha Indological Research Institute, 2025.

Appendixes

Appendix A

Atharva Veda 11.4 - Prāna Sukta, Oldest reference to prana and universal cycles

Homage to Prāna, him who hath dominion o'er the universe, Who hath become the Sovran Lord of all, on whom the whole depends!

Homage, O Prāna, to thy roar, to thunder-peal and lightning flash! Homage, O Prāna, unto thee what time thou sendest down thy rain!

When Prāna with a thunderous voice shouts his loud message to the plants, They straightway are impregnate, they conceive, and bear abundantly.

When the due season hath arrived and Prāna shouteth to herbs, then all is joyful, yea, each thing upon the surface of the earth.

When Prāna hath poured down his flood of rain upon the mighty land. Cattle and beasts rejoice thereat: Now great will he our strength, they cry.

Watered by Prāna's rain the plants have raised their voices in accord: Thou hast prolonged our life, they say, and given fragrance to us all.

Homage to thee when coming nigh, homage to thee departing hence! Homage, O Prāna, be to thee when standing and when sitting still.

Homage to thee at every breath thou drawest in and sendest forth! Homage to thee when turned away, homage to thee seen face to face! This reverence be to all of thee!

Prāna, communicate to us thy dear, thy very dearest form. Whatever healing balm thou hast, give us thereof that we may live.

Prāna robes living creatures as a father his beloved son. Prāna is sovran Lord of all, of all that breathes not, all that breathes

Prāna is Fever, he is Death. Prāna is worshipped by the Gods.

Prāna sets in the loftiest sphere the man who speaks the words of truth.

Prāna is Deshtri, and Virāj Prāna is reverenced by all. He is the Sun, he is the Moon. Prāna is called Prajāpati.

Both breaths are rice and barley, and Prāna is called the toiling ox: In barley is the inbreath laid, and rice is named the outward breath.

The human infant in the womb draws vital breath and sends it Lout: When thou, O Prāna, quickenest the babe it springs anew to life.

The name of Prāna is bestowed on Mātarisvan and on Wind. On Prāna, past and future, yea, on Prāna everything depends.

All herbs and plants spring forth and grow when thou, O Prāna quickenest, Plants of Atharvan, Angiras, plants of the deities and men.

When Prāna hath poured down his flood of rain upon the mighty earth, The plants are wakened into life, and every herd that grows on ground.

The man who knows this truth of thee, O Prāna, and what bears thee up To him will all present their gift of tribute in that loftiest will all present their gift of tribute in that loftiest world.

As all these living creatures are thy tributaries, Prāna, so Shall they bring tribute unto him who hears thee with attentive ears.

Filled with a babe, mid deities he wanders: grown; near at hand, he springs again to being. That Father, grown the present and the future, hath past into the son with mighty powers.

Hansa, what time he rises up, leaves in the flood one foot un-moved. If he withdrew it there would be no more tomorrow or to-day, Never would there be night, no more would daylight shine or morning flush.

It rolleth on, eight-wheeled and single-fellied, and with a thousand eyes, forward and backward. With one half it engendered all creation. What sign is there to tell us of the other?

Homage, O Prāna unto thee armed with swift bow among the rest, In whose dominion is this All of varied sort that stirs and works!

May he who rules this Universe of varied sort, that stirs and works, Prāna, alert and resolute, assist me through the prayer I pray.

Erect among the sleepers he wakes, and is never laid at length, No one hath ever heard that he hath been asleep while others slept.

Thou, Prāna, never shalt be hid, never shalt be estranged from me. I bind thee on myself for life, O Prāna, like the Waters' germ.

Translated by Ralph T.H. Griffith, 1895.

Appendix B
Chapter 7 of the Svaccanda Tantra

The following translation of the 7th chapter of the Svaccanda Tantra is not designed to be a critical edition, nor a literal translation of the verses. The tantric text is dense and at times speaks in code. In order to facilitate the understanding of the text I have tried to balance between a more literal translation when it was suited, to a more contextual one where I found the verses were too cryptic to be understood without deep commentary. For the professional this might be jarring, but for the lay reader this should make the text much more intelligible.

O Lord Maheśvara, by Your grace I have come to know about action (kriyā). Now, O Lord of the gods, kindly explain the divisions of Time in detail. (1)

O dear one, know that Time is of two types: solar (external) and spiritual (internal). It is favorable when there is a good weekday, proper planetary alignment, an auspicious time, and a good day. (2)

The waning and waxing of light indicate the southern and northern courses (dakṣiṇāyana and uttarāyaṇa). Eclipses of the Sun and Moon, as well as the seasons, are also manifestations of Time. (3)

The fortnight (pakṣa), month (māsa), hour (velā), equinoxes, and transitions between zodiac signs — All these are termed "solar" (external) time, O goddess, which brings merit or demerit. (4)

Now, O Devi, listen as I explain the internal or spiritual dimension of time. The human body is made up of six sheaths, comprising the five great elements and their subtle aspects. (5)

This body is governed by the mind, intellect, ego, the faculties of knowledge and action, All elements (tattvas), and deities, forming the complete embodied being. (6)

Within the body resides the Self and the sovereign life-energy (prāṇa), which moves through the nāḍīs. It is located primarily from the navel downward, extending to the root of the reproductive organs. (7)

From the center of the navel region, nāḍīs (subtle channels) extend in all directions—upwards, downwards, and sideways—like spokes of a wheel. Of these, ten are considered principal. (8)

From the ten primary nāḍīs, 72,000 subtle channels arise. These in turn give rise to more nāḍīs, and so on, in a branching, expansive system. (9)

It is said that the number of nāḍīs is as vast as the hair follicles on the body—just like a leaf is densely filled with fine threads or veins throughout. (10)

The bodies of all beings are likewise filled with nāḍīs, which are always filled with air and constantly circulate the life-force (ātma-śakti). (11)

They differ in their functions and paths of movement, And based on those differences, they are known by various names, O beautiful one. (12)

There are thousands of variations of the nāḍīs and their winds (vāyus), But ten nāḍīs are considered principal, O graceful one. (13)

Among them, O goddess of the gods, dwell the vital airs (vāyus). Listen now to the names and functions of these nāḍīs and their winds. (14)

They are: iḍā, piṅgalā, suṣumnā, gāndhārī, hastijihvā, pūṣā, yaśasvinī, (15) alambusā, kuhū, and śaṃkhinī — these are the ten major nāḍīs. They are the pathways of prāṇa (life-force) and the main conduits. (16)

The ten vāyus (vital airs) are: prāṇa, apāna, samāna, udāna, vyāna, nāga, kūrma, kṛkara, devadatta, and dhanañjaya. (17)

The nāḍīs and vital airs are arranged like a wheel, O beloved; one who moves through them attains success and yoga, O beautiful-faced one. (18)

O exaulted lady, in the repetition of mantras (japa), success comes through mastering them. Among the ten, three nāḍīs are most significant, O goddess. (19)

Two are said to be of bindu and nāda, and in the middle is śakti; in the heart chakra, these are described as beneficial for practitioners. (20)

Prāṇa indeed moves in them, according to the division of day and night. Thus, having clearly distinguished (its course), I will explain it to you. (21)

Impelled by the supreme power (śakti), established in the winds, prāṇa, and the Self. These three (prāṇa, ātman, and śakti), though indivisible, circulate everywhere. (22)

As they flow upward and downward through all the nāḍīs, they manifest as various functions and forms, of the sounds and letters. (23)

Among the 72,000 nāḍīs, ten principal ones emerge, and from the fundamental root—koṭi-dhātu, the primordial center—one supreme channel is established. (24)

The life-force, made of prāṇa and apāna, governs the processes of inhalation and exhalation. It is ever active in the chest region of all beings. (25)

Since it brings life (prāṇana), it is known as prāṇa. Now I shall describe to you the flow of day and night within prāṇa. (26)

The Sixteen tuṭis (smallest units of time, about 29.6 microseconds) have already been mentioned as measures of prāṇa. They are called "lavās" (fractions of time) when measured externally. (27)

In prāṇa every group of four tuṭis forms one yāma (a quarter of the day/ night), O goddess. Four yāmas thus make one day, using the same measure, O Devi. (28)

Likewise, four make up the night. Thus, eight yāmas form a full day-night cycle (ahorātra). Śiva is the haṃsa in dharma; the Sun is the haṃsa endowed with radiance. (29)

The soul (ātman) is referred to as "Haṁsa" (I am That), and prāṇa is connected to this Haṁsa. From it, time and the rising of the planets come into being. (30)

The constellations, zodiacal signs, stars, and their degrees all arise in prāṇa within the day-night cycle, O noble one. (31)

Now I will describe how the day-night cycle is measured within the body, based on the movement of prāṇa between the heart and the throat. (32)

The first prahara (quarter of day) is from the heart to one finger-breadth below the throat. The second is from there upward, reaching the mid-palate — that is the midday. (33)

At that time, homa (ritual offering), japa (chanting), and meditation are highly effective for liberation. From the nostrils to three finger-widths upward is the next span, O faithful one. (34)

This defines the third prahara, O beautiful lady. And up to the end of śakti (the uppermost point) is the fourth — this is considered the full day. (35)

When the fourth prahara ends, the inner 'sun' of prāṇa sets. This produces the twilight interval (sandhyā), lasting half a subtle time-unit (tuṭi). (36)

After this short pause, the flow begins again downward — This marks the moonrise, O goddess, and thus the night begins. (37)

Following the same order, prāṇa descends through the nocturnal watches. When it reaches the palate-region, midnight occurs, and the cycle continues in its patterned progression. (38)

When prāṇa reaches the heart-lotus again, that marks the early dawn. after half a tuṭi, O graceful one, the morning sandhyā occurs. (39)

And from that moment, the inner sunrise once more unfolds. In this same patterned order the prāṇic cycle endlessly repeats. (40)

The Sun moves during the day and the Moon within the flowing current of prāṇa. This combined inner sunrise and moonrise, I have now explained. (41)

Likewise, the planets starting with Mars (bhauma) move in proper sequence. All of them rise within the prāṇa — during each prahar (quarter of day/night), O dear one. (42)

A planet's 'day' corresponds to two praharas of prāṇic motion. Rāhu follows the lunar current; Ketu moves in the solar current. (43)

The planetary powers correspond symbolically to nāgas, the eight directional guardians, the eight forms of manifestation, and the eight lords of the Gaṇas. (44)

These cosmic groups correspond to the Rudras, the eight yogic powers, and the eight Vidyeśvaras (lords of mantra-knowledge), ranging from Ananta to Śikhaṇḍin. (45)

All levels of reality, from the highest transcendent down to the manifest tattvas, including the eight Bhairavas earlier described, are integrated within this cosmic order. (46)

These deities and principles, presiding over the planets and stars, Cause their rising and setting in conjunction with zodiac signs and lunar mansions (nakṣatras through the cycles of day and night. (47)

At midday and midnight, a special rise known as Abhijit occurs. Practices undertaken at this time yield the results sought by the sādhaka. (48)

So far, I have described to you the division of day and night. Now, I shall speak of fortnights, months, and years. (49)

Through the inner day and night, the outer time unit called kāṣṭhā is measured. Likewise through the inner month, the outer unit called kalā is established. (50)

O graceful one, thirty such inner days make one month. And twelve such months define one ghaṭikā. (51)

Three hundred and sixty day-nights constitute the year; this corresponds outwardly to the ghaṭikā. (52)

Sixty ghaṭikās that flow in one outer day and night when mapped onto the inner cycle become sixty years of prāṇic time. (53)

Now I shall describe for you the count of prāṇas, O radiant lady. There are 621,000 prāṇas in a day and night. (54)

This number (621,000) relates to the outer day but refers to the inner realm (adhyātma). Every seeker should know this count of prāṇas. (55)

He who remains absorbed in the sound of the "Haṁsa" prāṇa — the breath of the Self — Is the true knower of the supreme reality; the japa (repetition) of this sound grants both success and liberation. (56)

When prāṇa descends to the heart one gains yogic powers (siddhi); when it ascends beyond, merging with the supreme tattva, liberation arises. (57)

Even when the mind wanders and the senses are distracted, the prāṇa continues its natural rhythm effortlessly and without interruption. (58)

No agent produces or restrains it; the natural mantra haṃsa is spontaneously recited by the breath that dwells in the heart of all creatures. (59)

Thus, I have described to how inner prāṇic time expands into month and year. Next, I shall speak of lunar and solar eclipses. (60)

The prāṇic day-night cycle forms the basis for the waxing and waning fortnights. I will now show how this extends into the full lunar month. (61)

The half-tuṭis (smallest time units) above and below are called the pause (rest). The fifteen tuṭis in the middle correspond to the lunar days (tithis) of the month. (62)

"From the heart as the starting point, the rising half-tuṭi marks the onset of day. The subsequent half-tuṭi marks the emergence of night. (63)

All celestial patterns—zodiac, planets, stars—mirror their ordered rising within the internal prāṇic day-night cycle. (64)

Fifteen tuṭis form one fortnight (pakṣa). If there is a break in a tithi (if a tithi, i.e. lunar day lasts less than one solar day), it is to be understood as a loss (inauspicious for activity); if a tithi grows (lasts more than 2 solar days), it signifies gain (extremely auspicious). (65)

(in the breath cycle) a break in a tithi is marked by a cough while a sigh (or long exhale) is the inner expanded tithi. When the prāṇa flows upward during the dark fortnight (kṛṣṇa pakṣa), dissolution and withdrawal happen. (66)

Harsh or fierce actions performed during this time can lead to success. However, auspicious deeds during the dark fortnight generally do not yield fruit, O virtuous one. (67)

The final tuṭi where śakti fully enters into prāṇa at the culmination of contraction, this point corresponds internally to the Amāvasyā new-moon moment of the dark fortnight, O lovely lady. (68)

That half-tuṭi located in the middle and upper region of śakti is called the junction of fortnights — the transition between Amāvasyā and Pratipadā (first day of bright half). (69)

When the tithi is interrupted, the inner analogy to a solar eclipse manifests: the lunar principle overshadows the solar one. (70)

Within that overlap, Rāhu, the seeker of ambrosia (amṛta), devours the nectar secreted by the Moon. (71)

After drinking, he releases the orb; then he is said to be freed. This is known in the world as the solar eclipse. (72)

When Rāhu, the Sun, and the Moon all appear aligned in one straight conjunction, Then a great eclipse (mahāgrahaṇa) occurs. (73)

That time is considered extremely sacred for all beings. Bathing, charity, worship, homa (offerings), and japa (chanting) done then bear immense fruit. (74)

What practitioners perform then yields infinite fruit; and after leaving that half-tuṭi, the bright fortnight begins. (75)

With the beginning of the bright fortnight, śakti manifests creative power from her womb below; from there growth follows, making this period ideal for auspicious undertakings. (76)

When a practitioner realizes the haṃsa nature of prāṇa and aligns with the initial downward phase, meditative and mantra-based practices unfailingly bear fruit. (77)

Signs of the zodiac, planets, constellations (ṛkṣas), yogas and karaṇas (astrological components) All arise during the day and night according to the cycle described previously. (78)

The cycle renews itself exactly as before. The first tithi, Pratipat, corresponds to the Moon possessing a single kalā—the first increment of luminosity. (79)

On the second, the second tithi; it increases gradually. The tithis proceed thus up to the fifteenth tuṭi. (The lunar growth continues step by step, with each tuṭi corresponding to a tithi, until it reaches the full-moon level at the fifteenth). (80)

A sādhaka must recognize the full-moon phase, for it is the moment when ritual, mantra-practice, and meditation yield their fullest results. (81)

On that (tithi) the Moon becomes full, O beautiful-eyed one; and the half-tuṭi belonging to it is known as the fortnight junction. (82)

Half of the full moon tithi merges with the first half of the next day (pratipad). At the center of the heart-lotus (hṛtpadma), this is where the lunar eclipse is said to occur. (83)

Just as in the outer world a lunar eclipse occurs apart from the sun, so within the yogic body the same principle applies. At that moment, practices such as meditation, mantra recitation, and offerings generate exceptional merit. (84)

O Goddess, in both fortnights there is eclipse of moon and sun; this indeed grants various siddhis to the disciplined practitioner. (85)

When the yogin transcends the dual motion of waxing and waning (the internal lunar cycle), using the earlier-taught yogic method, he reaches the state conducive to liberation. (86)

Abandoning all that is below, and establishing oneself steadily in unmanī (a meditative state beyond mind), One should focus entirely on meditation, holding onto the Supreme Inner Movement. (87)

There is no doubt of his liberation; otherwise he attains only siddhis. For all embodied beings, eclipses occur in both fortnights. (88)

Thus this has been told, O beautiful-faced one, concerning the inner day and night lasting as long as life. Now the cycle of the year is described. (89)

The internal zodiac is laid out within the upper body, beginning at the heart and ascending upward. Each of the six rāśis occupies six finger-widths along the central channel. (90)

Within each of the six-aṅgula rāśis, five subtle tithis are mapped. Each tithi is divided into a 'day' and 'night' portion in the inner yogic cycle. (91)

These six sets of five tithis are the monthly day-nights; by these thirty day-nights the two-fortnight month is said to arise. (92)

In the internal zodiacal cycle, the transition corresponding to Capricorn (Makara) is located at the heart, where prāṇa reverses direction and begins its ascent.(93)

The subtle zodiac progresses upward: from Capricorn to Aquarius (Kumbha) after six aṅgulas, then into Pisces (Mīna) after rising two aṅgulas above he throat region.

From above the throat to the end of the palate, the transition occurs into Aries (Meṣa). Up to the tip of the nose, the transition covers six finger-widths (95)

This is the transition point of Viṣuva (the equinox), located in the northern path (uttarayāṇa). It is especially potent for japa, homa, worship, and meditation — all leading to great spiritual results. (96)

Leaving behind the tip of the nose, the vital breath (prāṇa haṃsa) moves in the sign of Taurus (Vṛṣabha). Leaving behind six more finger-widths, it transitions again into Gemini (Mithuna). (97)

Up to the endpoint of Śakti (end of the reach of the breath 12 fingers beyond the nose), the pathway of energy is known as the transition in Gemini. From Capricorn to the end of Gemini, O noble one, this is known as the Uttarāyaṇa (northern journey). (98)

The northern ascent (uttarāyaṇa) within the body is for supra-mundane attainment, not for worldly siddhis. In this region, acts such as ritual bathing, meditation, dāna, pūjā, homa, and japa shine with special potency. (99)

Even if these acts are performed thousands of times by practitioners, they don't yield worldly rewards in this birth — But their results will surely manifest in the next world (afterlife). (100)

As the internal solar path ascends from Makara to Mithuna, the subtle days (inner light-phases) grow. In this phase, the yogin should gather and restrain the vīrya—the vital lunar-solar essence—since this is the period governing growth throughout the cosmos. (101)

The haṃsa-prāṇa draws the subtle essence into the 'womb'. This essence, bearing countless subtle forms and impressions accumulated over ages, is gathered inward for refinement.(102)

After the ascent, the cycle reverses from Cancer (Karkaṭa), all is again showered (as in rainfall or blessing); Hence, beginning with Capricorn, one should practice meditation, offerings, and mantra recitation. (103)

These practices yield fruits in the next world (paraloka). Any purascaraṇa (preparatory practices) and mantra vow (vrata) undertaken at that time become extremely potent. (104)

From Pisces (Mīna) onward, one should begin all practices for attaining mantra perfection (mantrasiddhi). Even externally in the world, trees respond in alignment with the six seasons. (105)

Like Flower Blossoms bring joy, lit by the God of Love (Kāmadeva) armed with flowers; Mantras, aligned with time and seasonal discipline, are activated accordingly. (106)

Ignited with knowledge-insight, producing siddhi and liberation, these mantra have the nature of the inner spiritual sound, they are stirred by the 'tasting' of the six emotional-energetic rasas (flavors) within the yogic experience. (107)

When prāṇa rises to the Mīna-point (located at the throat), haṃsa-awareness illumines perception. At this stage, subtle inner sound (nāda) becomes distinctly perceptible. (108)

From that point onward, japa proceeds smoothly; O Goddess, at the end of Gemini (Mithuna), siddhi (spiritual attainment) arises. (109)

When the prāṇa descends from bindu-śakti, oriented downward through the channels of siddhi, it 'rains' its essence beginning in Karkaṭa and continuing through Tulā (mapped internally through the palate). (110)

As the prāṇa descends again below the throat and spreads from the heart-lotus, the yogin must engage in practice to stabilize inner realization (ātma-siddhi) and for vitality (puṣṭi). (111)

In the descending solar path (dakṣiṇāyana) creation (sṛṣṭi) occurs. The haṃsa, moving under Śakti within the heart center, enters the internal zodiacal point corresponding to Cancer (Karkaṭa). (112)

After leaving six finger-widths behind, it again transitions in Leo (Siṃha); Leaving another six finger-widths, it transitions again into Virgo (Kanyā). (113)

The passage from the nose-tip down to the palate marks the internal southern equinox, this is the Libra transition called the southern equinox (Dakṣiṇa Viṣuva). (114)

Any practice performed during this time yields worldly desires in this life; It conquers death, brings peace and nourishment — hence one should begin spiritual effort then. (115)

Therefore, one who takes six-flavored food (ṣaḍrasāhāra) will nourish the body below the throat; Leaving six finger-widths behind, the prāṇa transitions into Scorpio (Vṛścika) again. (116)

Leaving two aṅgulas above the throat and four below, leaving Scorpio, the transit into Sagittarius is said to occur. (117)

From six finger-widths below, the being moves in Sagittarius at the heart center; After passing through the heart-lotus (hṛtpadma), the Haṃsa (soul) rises upward again. (118)

The entire twelve-sign cycle within the subtle body maps the full cycle of embodied life. The upward and downward movements of prāṇa constitute the internal year, determining vitality and longevity. (119)

Worldly and otherworldly attainments — lower, middle, and higher — Have now been described through the two solstices (ayanas); but liberation comes only by transcending both. (120)

Remaining in unmanī (mind-transcending state) beyond both solstices, One who abides there and performs japa and meditation attains liberation (mokṣa). (121)

Once liberation is attained, there is no return — this is the vow (pratijñā) of Bhairava. Now, O radiant one, listen to the cycle of twelve years (dvādaśābdodaya). (122)

The outer year begins with Caitra; similarly, the inner twelve-year cycle has its own starting point aligned with that rhythm. Mantra-practice should be synchronized to this cosmological beginning (123)

O beautiful one, the twelve-year cycle should be understood as beginning from Caitra; Now I shall describe its characteristics and how prāṇa is divided within it. (124)

There, each year is divided into a symbolic day and night, as previously stated; Each year consists of twelve divisions (āṃśas), O dear one. (125)

The twelve day-nights form the twelve-year period; multiplying them by five produces the twelve-year season. (126)

Doubling that, the time-unit is established; tripling it gives the ayana; and six times that gives the year. (127)

The twelve transits here, as described in the preivous section, become the years in the twelve-year rising of prāṇa. (128)

Now hear from me the total number of days and nights in the twelve-year cycle: They number 4,320 (four thousand three hundred twenty). (129)

O Goddess, I have thus explained the twelve-year rise (dvādaśābdodaya) through prāṇa; Now I shall speak to you of the sixty-year cycle (ṣaṣṭyabdodaya), right here again. (130)

The sixty-year cycles beginning with Ānanda are to be known, O beautiful-faced one; they occur in the prāṇa that moves downward and upward, within the one prāṇa, O divine beauty. (131)

They move in divisions; thus I shall explain them. He who worships the mantra beginning with Ānanda, O Goddess... (132)

For that person, bliss arises along with the mantra, O goddess of the gods. In twelve years, the day and night are divided into five parts. (133)

In the sixty-year cycle, five day-night phases are mentioned. When multiplied by six, one month is constituted. (134)

With those twelve, one year is formed, O Goddess. This measure is declared as one and five-twelfths of an aṅgula. (135)

With six finger-units, five years are formed; sixty years arise from them. From the heart lotus upward to the power of Śakti, thirty years manifest (in the body). (136)

From Śakti down to the heart lotus, thirty years also manifest. I shall now state the count of day-nights in the sixty-year cycle. (137)

There are twenty-one thousand six hundred (21,600) day-nights in the sixty years, O lovely-faced one. (138)

The sixty-year cycle has been described as resting in one prāṇa. This also applies during lunar and solar eclipses, fortnights, months, and solstices. (139)

It applies at the beginnings and ends of yugas, and also within a year. And within the twelve-year period and the sixty-year cycle, O beautiful one. (140)

Whatever actions are performed in the external time — through bathing, giving, sacrifices, worship, offerings, japa, or knowledge and yoga... (141)

The great result of those actions, O rising one, is obtained by the one who knows and honors (i.e aligns with) the movement of the prāṇahaṃsa. (142)

Its movement becomes self-experienced and clear through mastery over the nāḍī system; or else, even through intense practice of japa alone. (143)

The mantra-practitioner knows yoga, and knowing thus, attains omniscience. I will again explain this cycle according to the division of the three nāḍīs. (144)

In the southern and northern transits and in the equinoctial movement—this is how the haṃsa moves in this world of moving and unmoving beings. (145)

Dwelling within as time itself, shaping the world through kalās, supported by the three nāḍīs, it is established in the three paths. (146)

Operating through the triple guṇa (sattva, rajas, tamas), the three states (jāgrat, svapna, suṣupti), the six forms of causality, and the three primordial Śaktis (icchā, jñāna, kriyā). (147)

permeated by the three shaktis cchā-jñāna-kriyā , situated between moon, sun, and fire: the nāḍī called Piṅgalā is said to be in the right nostril. (148)

Iḍā is in the left, and Suṣumnā is established in the middle. The right path is the way of the gods; the left is the path of the ancestors. (149)

The middle path is the path of Śiva; one who enters it is not born again. The right corresponds to the waking state and sattva, the left to the dream state and rajas. (150)

The middle is to be known as tamas and the state of deep sleep. Brahmā and Īśvara dwell on the right; on the left, Viṣṇu and Sadāśiva. (151)

In the center are Rudra and Śiva — and beyond all is Paraśiva, the transcendental. In the right is Jñāna shakti (knowledge), in the left is Kriyā shakti (action), and in the center is supreme will. (152)

Raudrī (fierce śakti) and icchā (will) dwell in the center; the supreme śakti is both transcendent and immanent. The Sun is situated on the right; the Moon shines on the left. (153)

Fire is in the center, illuminating and ripening all things. It digests everything arising from the qualities of the Moon and others. (154)

By its own power, it reveals the supreme, flawless Reality. All the zodiac signs, planets, constellations, and yogas... (155)

They all move in succession along the paths of the Moon and Sun. The Sun and Moon consume them all, one after the other, O dear one. (156)

Endowed with the essences of Moon and Sun, they are established in the three paths. The Sun heats, the Moon pours nectar. (157)

The whole universe is of lunar-solar nature; the solar path on the right is called the northern course. (158)

The left, lunar side is the southern course. The lunar-solar equinox arises from the two nostril-channels (flowing equally). (159)

There are five northern transits, five southern transits, and between the two, the two equinoctial transits. (160)

The solar southern path (Piṅgalā) gives success in abhicāra (rituals for control, hostile magic, etc.); the northern lunar path (Iḍā) is for increase, nourishment, and pacification rites. (161)

When the prāṇa moves from the southern to the northern direction or vice versa, it is termed the inner solstice (Saṅkrānti). (162)

When prāṇa shifts from the southern nāḍī (Piṅgalā) to the northern (Iḍā), remaining in the middle for half a duration, the ascent begins. This is the threshold of inner uttarāyaṇa. (163)

That point is known as the Viṣuvat (equinox). When the prāṇa moves from northern to southern course, that is the transition to Dakṣiṇāyana. (164)

As long as it flows half there and half in the southern side, that is the southern equinox, arising in the southern course. (165)

Worship, japa, homa, and other acts done during this time become liberating. A Guru can liberate the disciple who is situated in this state through meditative yoga. (166)

Externally in day and night, and internally in the subtle body, O beautiful one, the life-breath (Haṁsa) transitions through twenty-four Saṅkrāntis (transitions between zodiacs). (167)

Twelve are said to occur during the day, and twelve during the night. One equinox is in the morning, the second at midday. (168)

The third occurs in the afternoon, and the fourth at midnight. These four transitions per day and night are known to bring liberation. (169)

The twenty-four transits arise naturally from the balanced flow; the haṃsa ever carries nine hundred (breaths) one after another. (170)

This is the measurement described. If it moves otherwise, it should be observed whether the effect is auspicious or inauspicious. (171)

Whether for oneself or another, the yogi should determine this. When the eastern rise of the sun occurs, O beautiful one— (172)

He should examine life(span) and (approaching)death at that moment. The yogi, with a well-controlled mind, seated in the yogic posture— (173)

Remembering (keeping) his prāṇa within the suṣumnā, he should remain very tranquil, with mind absorbed in the single prāṇa. (174)

When the breath is stable in Piṅgalā, and then shifts toward the equinox-point, then the yogin, examining time should determine the prognostic outcome. (175)

A single day-night (inhale exhale cycle) signifies one year of life remaining, O noble lady. Two days and nights correspond to two years of life. (176)

Three years remaining is dignified by three day-night units, four years by four such, five years by five, and six years by six. (177)

Seven years by seven days, eight by eight, nine by nine, ten by ten days. (178)

Eleven years by eleven days, and twelve years by twelve days, O beloved. (179)

By movement during seven Yāmas (7/8th of an inhale exhale cycle), one lives for six months. By six Prahars (6/8th of an inhale exhale cycle) , he lives for three months. (180)

With five Prahars, life is one and a half months; with four, he lives one month, O goddess. (181)

With three Prahars, half a month is attained; with two, eight days of life remain. (182)

With one (internal) Prahar (i.e. 1/8 of a breath or very shallow), one lives for one (external) prahar (i.e. 1/8th of a day or 3 hours); if only one Prahar passes, then half of that yields two Prahars of life. (183)

If the breath becomes chaotic, flowing simultaneously or erratically through all three channels (iḍā, piṅgalā, suṣumnā), it is a sign of imminent death. The yogin should immediately diagnose the exact moment. (184)

From that day onward, the month, fortnight, day, and year should be precisely noted and the determination made carefully. (185)

In the time of the northern course this has been taught to you. But even when the breath is disturbed or unbalanced, the signs of death can still be read. Listen to this further teaching. (186)

When, with the thumb placed at the ear-aperture, he does not hear the inner sound, his death should be predicted within six months, O Goddess. (187)

When he does not hear the supreme sound within the hum, like the "Cīra" or "Ciñciṇī" chirping of cicadas – he will live for one month, O beloved. (188)

Hear from me the signs of uprooting, defect, and death-yoga: when the prāṇa carries the fivefold transit into the mouth-aperture– (189)

That is called the uprooting-yoga, it signifies: displacement from one's position, loss of wealth, anxiety, and increase of disease arise. (190)

Destruction of friends and home, and loss of radiance arise when the right nostril alone flows outside the proper southern course. (191)

With an eight-fold saṃkrānti (eight-step abnormal breath) creates the 'one-eye yoga' (disease-pattern) associated with bile and heat, reflected in eye disorders and. (192)

Pain, eruptions, suffering, and chest disorders arise when thirteen saṃkrāntis occur through the left nostril alone. (193)

Fever, headache, pain, piles, stiffness, painful urination, diabetes, and anemia arise. (194)

When prāṇa moves in Iḍā it aggravates phlegm-diseases. Whatever flow is observed, its effect appears at the same time the next day. (195)

He is afflicted by all diseases when the left alternates irregularly. Now another diagnostic based on touch (of the breath) below and above the nostril. (196)

When touched above, if the breath rises (if the breath touches the upper part of the nose), the previously mentioned disorders occur; when the right nostril flows, there is verbal abuse and harm. (197)

If it passes through the middle, one may attain superiority over others. If it moves here and there in many ways, yet through one passage— (198)

He will gain honor, many gifts, and rewards. When the Prāṇa Haṁsa moves slowly through the Suṣumnā— (199)

The prāṇa performs twelve transitions while reaching the equinox (viṣuva), and twelve more after it. This completes the full 24-saṃkrānti internal day-night cycle. (200)

When the number of prāṇa-transitions (saṃkrāntis) declines from the expected norm, the remaining lifespan shortens accordingly. A single reduction in the saṃkrānti-count equals the loss of one month of life. (201)

O beautiful one, one reduced saṃkrānti causes the loss of thirty (internal) prāṇas; which over thirty days manifests as a full month's reduction of lifespan. (202)

At the end of the month death occurs instantly, O lovely-faced one. Thus I have explained the death-yoga to you, O radiant one. (203)

Year, month, fortnight, tithi, and moment — whenever one practices, from that time onwards one should determine the corresponding time. (204)

The wise know prāṇa-movement through the paths of Iḍā and Suṣumnā; thus I have told you this auspicious teaching pertaining to the southern course. (205)

By diagnosing bodily (prāṇa-based) signs correctly, the yogin overcomes not only death but every form of misfortune. Prognosis becomes a gateway to mastery. (206)

Meditating on the Lord of Time, or the free-moving Haṁsa, or the Supreme Lord, established in the nasal passage, he can create and dissolve the universe. (207)

Remaining there he should contemplate all beings as abiding in That; meditating on That, he conquers death. (But) one should not imagine the formless as having a 'place,' O Lord. (208)

Through meditation for six months, omniscience arises; the yogi who unites with time understands all three dimensions of time. (209)

Reciting or meditating on the Kāla-Haṃsa, he becomes of the form of Time, O Goddess; he moves as Svacchanda, like Time itself. (210)

Having slain death, abandoning old age, free from disease and fear, he gains knowledge, distant hearing, thought-reading, and sight. (211)

From conquering Time he always attains all lordly qualities. Meditating in the right nostril he obtains Brahmā-like powers — mastery over creation, articulation, and manifestation. (212)

His life and vigor become equal to (that deity's); he knows the past. Meditating in the left nostril he knows the future and has the strength of Viṣṇu. (213)

Then he becomes a sovereign yogi equal to the divine, knowing past, present, and future entirely, arising from being in the middle path (suṣumnā). (214)

Always through meditation-yoga he attains equality with Rudra, equal to Him in lifespan, strength, vigor, form, and lordly power. (215)

By transcending Brahmā's nature one attains the lordly state; the sovereignty of Sadāśiva over Viṣṇu is attained by surpassing (Viṣṇu's) nature. (216)

Meditating on the state beyond Rudra, he becomes Śiva. Thus victory over death is known; triumph comes from meditating on amṛta (immortality). (217)

Meditate on the heart-lotus situated in the channel between the nāḍīs (suṣumnā), white, fully opened, with sixteen petals and endowed with sixteen kalās. (218)

Within it the full Moon shaped like the pericarp of a flowe, and in its center one should contemplate oneself, pure like flawless crystal. (219)

(This lotus is) Filled with waves of nectar from the sacred ocean of amṛta, and above it lies a second lotus in the great ocean of Śakti's nectar. (220)

This downward-facing lotus, has a full moon as its pericarp; in its center, visualize a swan (haṁsa) facing downward, crowned by a bindu flame. (221)

Raining divine nectar, contemplate it flowing everywhere, and visualize it entering through the upper opening of the Self. (222)

Visualize yourself bathed and filled with the dense, abundant white nectar that destroys death. (223)

Visualize the entire body filled with nectar, flowing through all the lotus-stem like nāḍī-openings. (224)

Thus, with constant union of the Self, one becomes equal to the Lord of Nectar; abandoning disease, death, and aging, one plays with yogic powers like aṇimā, etc. (225)

Through this meditation on nectar, one gains victory over time and death; or by remaining established in the supreme reality, one is unaffected by all times. (226)

Meditate on the supreme reality, free from temporal movement, without stain or division, formless and beyond all measures. (227)

The partless Self is pure; the body is the impurity, joined with six causes and containing all tattvas. (228)

Color, bindu, sound, and the pervading power of Śakti, ending with the universal mind—all these form the foundation of impurity. (229)

The supreme Self is the true content; the state beyond that is called unmanā (mindless state), beyond which lies the supreme truth, free from all dualities. (230)

(Śiva is) All-pervading, auspicious in all directions, present within all things, facing all directions, based in the five sets of five principles (25 tattvas), endowed with eighteen qualities. (231)

If one realizes the supreme within this (everything), then one is freed from bondage; the causes, mantras, and kalās like nivṛtti, etc., are also transcended. (232)

Bindu, half-moon, the upward-rising restraining nāda, Śakti, the pervading one, the universal mind, and unmanā (levels of inner sound). (233)

This fivefold group of fives has been told to you, O beautiful one; now hear of the thirty-six tattvas and their qualities. (234)

Ego, intelligence, mind, sense objects, as well as the means of grasping, touching, and support and shakto, these are considered to be the eight. (235)

These eight qualities are the eightfold Bhairava; together with prāṇa-haṃsa and śakti they become the eighteen qualities. (236)

Beyond these lies the supreme Reality, not relying on articulation; free from syllable and non-syllable (beyond the levels of sound), the supreme unsyllabic Reality. (237)

How can there be liberation in letters? How can space hold a flower? As long as speech expresses it, or it is written— (238)

As long as (speech persists) he is known as sakala (with attributes); the niṣkala is without distinction, free from creation and dissolution, free from action and time. (239)

By downward movement there is creation; by upward movement dissolution. By downward movement he is born; by upward movement he dies. (240)

Having abandoned impurity from birth and death, one should remain established in the mode of reality (tattva-vṛtti); and that mode of reality has been explained as free from all paths and limiting conditions. (241)

Freed from the properties of the paths of principles and from causes as well, the yogī established in the mode of reality is beyond all undertakings. (242)

Free from attachment and aversion, devoid of dejection and pleasure, he neither desires nor condemns, and never engages with objects of the senses. (243)

Equal toward enemy and friend, equal toward a brāhmaṇa and a dog-eater, he becomes one who sees equally at all times and remembers everything as permeated by Śiva. (244)

He should likewise always remember himself in this way, and all tattvas, beings, letters, and mantras. (245)

Through this Śiva-contemplation, they are always under his control; and he no longer performs merit or demerit, O virtuous one. (246)

Having done what was to be done, serene in self, he has no further duty; in this world and the next he is always completely fulfilled. (247)

Freed from dharma and adharma, merit and sin, he has no 'allowed or forbidden' food, nor any 'allowed or forbidden' drink. (248)

For him there is no impure and no pure, O virtuous one. He is ever without expectation, free from all dependence. (249)

He has no sacred field, no pilgrimage place, no observance, no restraint; his sacred field is the supreme Śakti from which everything arises. (250)

From her, O Goddess, all paths arise and move while abiding there; She is the supreme peaceful pilgrimage place, eternally pervaded by bliss. (251)

That by which this infinite universe is pervaded with its universal powers (Śiva)— knowing this, with constant dispassion toward saṃsāra, is called yama (the moral rules of restraint). (252)

Observance (niyama) is constant contemplation in the continuity of the supreme Reality; one should not conceive of self in terms of caste, family, or relatives. (253)

He should behave as belonging to all varṇas but not be bound by any; through constant contemplation of the Supreme, he abides in the supreme dharma. (254)

All-knowing, fully satisfied, complete by nature, autonomous, with unimpaired power, resting in the beginningless and endless. (255)

His awareness is beginningless and incomparable, free from time-divisions, free from movement and utterance, beyond day and night. (256)

He does not keep vigil by day nor sleep at night, abiding solely in his own nature, he is free from day and night. (257)

Thus the yogin lives, having attained equality with the Supreme. Time cannot reckon him, even in hundreds of millions of aeons. (258)

He is freed while living, who has this contemplation constantly. Śiva being continually contemplated—Time does not measure Śiva. (259)

The yogin, through the Svacchanda-yoga (freedom of will yoga) and moving with Svacchanda's freedom, being joined to the Svacchanda-state, attains equality with Svacchanda. (260)

Free, entirely free, he moves freely always. Thus have the death-signs and other omens been (also) described. (261)

The lordly yogin knows, through yoga, the signs that arise internally from nāda (internal sounds); conquering these by yoga according to the method taught. (262)

What the non-yogin or unpracticed one knows—these external signs, bodily omens—hear them from me. (263)

If the palate, lips, and throat become dry, if the complexion suddenly turns ashen, and if the shoulders appear broken or fallen, he will die within six months. (264)

He who sees daily a deep-blue circle in the sky, or white, green, or black, dies within half a year. (265)

If one sees the sun without rays, the moon without its marks, or the stars or moonlight as black, he has a lifespan of six months. (266)

He who sees in a dream a golden-colored man, tawny or black, lives only six months. (267)

He who sees his own shadow without a head lives six months. Likewise, dreams of being anointed with oil, of drinking, or of being adorned with red garlands and red unguents. (268)

When indeed he sees in a dream red garments and black ones, and (when he sees himself) surrounded by ghosts, piśācas, rakṣasas, dogs, cows, jackals, and boars. (269)

(Seeing himself) surrounded as he goes by vultures, crows, buffaloes, camels, and donkeys, and (seeing) the eating of limbs, being carried off, being naked, and exceedingly distressed. (270)

One who sees such (dreams) lives only for one year; (and if) the conch-like pulsation (micro-pulses) in the middle of the arm or in the vital ankle-joints ceases... (271)

He surely comes to death for whom those pulsations are not present, the same applies to the body's lunar and solar circles, at the Dhruva point, and at the Arundhatī point. (272)

note: *Traditional yogic physiology identifies certain micro-pulses as signs of life-force circulation. When these "śaṅkha-spandana" signs disappear, it means the nāḍīs have ceased carrying prāṇa to the limbs.*

The man who does not see the mahāyāna surely dies. The 'great path' is said to be the smoke arising in the aperture of the palate. (273)

The tongue is said to be Arundhatī; the tip of the nose is called Dhruva. The circle (seen) at the eye's end, covered by the eyelashes, is the orb of the moon and sun. (274)

If one does not see this even in the outer sky, he surely dies. If he suddenly becomes fat or suddenly becomes emaciated— (275)

—excessively angry or excessively fearful, he lives one year. Seeing in a dream a black man clothed in black, wielding an iron staff— (276)

—approaching him, his lifespan is three months. He whose heart dries (feels dry) immediately after bathing— (277)

—and whose limbs become cold—he lives for one season. Seeing a bow at night, a meteor by day, lightning in a cloudless sky— (278)

—or the heat coming from all direction, even in an unburned place—he lives one month. He whose eyes constantly discharfe (fluid) and who cannot hear sounds clearly— (279)

For whom the face is like a red lotus, and the tongue is black—(280)

When various discolorations appear on the body, and when the heart of a person trembles, and when there is trembling of the palate and also of the navel, he lives only half a month. (281)

When a man with contracted nostrils does not smell the smoke of a lamp, and does not recognize what he saw earlier, he lives four months. (282)

He who does not see the bindu, which constantly in front of the face and is beneficial, and who constantly suffers from hiccups, lives for one year. (283)

These external marks and bodily death-omens, O beloved, can be counteracted by worship, mantra-recitation, fire-offering, meditation, and concentration. (284)

By performing the protective rites they are overcome—there is no doubt. But how is the purification of the nāḍīs and the mastery of the vital winds to be accomplished? (285)

Tell me, O Lord, its place, its form, its sound, and its method—the supreme essence of yoga, more secret than the secret, O beloved. (286)

Hear that yoga which has not been told to anyone, in its true form. (It should be practiced) in an excellent, auspicious place on earth, not near fire or water. (287)

In a place free from sand and gravel, free from dry trees, silent, devoid of insects and anthills, and protected from dangers. (288)

In a holy place, in the company of the virtuous, there he should practice yoga, having worshipped the God of gods, Bhairava, along with Vināyaka. (289)

Having bowed to the former teachers, disciplined and devoted to meditation, he should assume svastika-āsana, or padma-āsana, or the auspicious posture. (290)

With a supportive half-moon-shaped yoga-strap, arranged as comfortable, having performed the burning and cleansing (rites), he should moisten it with nectar. (291)

With external and internal rites he should accomplish the unification; then the internal worship is to be performed as before, and the supreme (worship) likewise. (292)

He should practice the free-moving haṃsa through the yogic path in ten ways, (uttering) the mantra that transcends the bindu and has the form of light at the end of nāda. (293)

Having conceived the object of meditation beyond conceptualization, one should meditate by that which pervades all; one should inhale through the left nostril and exhale through the right. (294)

This nāḍī-purification belongs to the path of liberation; prāṇāyāma is known as threefold: exhalation, inhalation, and retention. (295)

These are the external general (methods); again, internally there are three. By the internal method he should exhale and inhale. (296)

Having performed motionless retention, the three internal acts are to be done: leading the mind from the navel to the heart and away from the sphere of the senses. (297)

The fourth prāṇāyāma is said to be exceedingly peaceful. When the restraint of prāṇa is complete, having brought it to the navel, one should then exhale properly. (298)

Slowly he should release the breath through the left nostril. The Air concentration is in the thumb center (where the soul, the size of a thumb resides, i.e. the heart), and the Fire concentration is at the center of the navel. (299)

The solar concentration is in the throat region, and the water concentration is located at the uvula. The Ether-concentration at the crown of the head is said to produce all accomplishments. (300)

With practices elevated in counts of one, two, three, four, and five, it becomes perfected. When prāṇa is fully restrained, it goes to the crown of the head and then returns. (301)

That is called udghāta and should always be known by yogīs; attachment and aversion are abandoned through well-sustained prāṇāyāma. (302)

By concentrations one burns sin; in pratyāhāra there is restraint of the senses; At the heart-knot, the navel, the throat, and at all vital joints likewise (these practices are applied). (303)

Prāṇa and the other vāyus are established thus; hear from me their form and sound. One is like a quick, high note, red in color, resembling the indragopa insect. (304)

The forms of the five (vāyus) are also like milk and like crystal. Their sounds are sweet like bells or bronze, like the call of an elephant, a great resonant sound. (305)

The sound of the five vāyus beginning with prāṇa is described as follows: murmuring, laughter, song, dance, and the movement or noise of battle—these are its modes. (306)

All crafts and activities are the functioning of prāṇa itself. It brings food and drink into the body and causes their waste to be expelled downward. (307)

Apāna causes blindness and ear-disease; samāna brings equality to what is eaten, licked, and drunk. (308)

Agitation, hiccups, and sneezing are the activity of udāna; sweat, horripilation, pain, burning, and aching of the limbs (are also its effects). (309)

These are the functions of vyāna, and one perceives touch through it. It is situated in the thumb, the knee, the heart, the eyes, and in the head. (310)

Nāga and the other (subsidiary vāyus) have many forms; learn from me their actions: producing delight, agitation, drying, and fear. (311)

Nāga, Kūrma, Kṛkara, Devadatta, and the fifth, Dhanañjaya; another causes deep sleep, and another unites (the body)—these are the subsidiary vāyus. (312)

Constriction and interruption of breath, gurgling, and the departure (of life)—these are the activities of the five Nāga and others at the time of death. (313)

Even at the time of departure, Dhanañjaya does not go away after the body is left. Kūrma contracts, and it dries up the body. (314)

One must first conquer prāṇa; when prāṇa is conquered, the mind is conquered. When the mind is conquered, the supreme truth becomes revealed. (315)

One should meditate on prāṇa and apāna at the perineal region, on prāṇa-samāna at the navel, on prāṇa-udāna at the throat, and on prāṇa-vyāna as pervading everywhere. (316)

One should restrain Nāga and the other vāyus, united with prāṇa, in their proper locations. And the duration of this restraint—I will now explain; listen to me. (317)

Beginning with a single time-beat, he should meditate upon it until it reaches five hundred. When the wind (prāṇa) is thus conquered, he becomes master of the acts of transition and ascent. (318)

Divine radiance, auspicious fragrance, and intelligence increase; divine sight and hearing arise, and divine speech is born. (319)

Like the wind he may move through the worlds; he sees the siddhas and the gods. Whatever is thought in the mind is obtained; the eight qualities arise. (320)

He becomes fully fulfilled in all desires, free from all dualities, released from the bondage of saṃsāra, and becomes equal to Śiva. (321)

When prāṇa and apāna are united in the short measure, at the navel-base there arise sweating and trembling, O lord of yogis. (322)

Then again one should restrain prāṇa and apāna at the heart; through the long-duration practice, at that very moment he may fall upon the ground. (323)

Similarly, restrain prāṇa in the throat. By the long-duration practice, the dream-state then arises. (324)

At the eyebrow-center, through union with the bindu, he should effect the restraint of prāṇa. There deep sleep arises, and after a moment he awakens again. (325)

Taking refuge at the crown-gate, begin the partless meditation; by such practice, inner certainty then arises for him. (326)

When the cranial gate is being pierced, there is a sensation like an ant's thorn. Breaking through all the stages gradually, he reaches those culminating in unmanī (beyond thought). (327)

With the signs described before, O Goddess, he attains spontaneity. The state of unmanas indeed arises for the practitioner in this very body. (328)

He may move into other bodies and is not afflicted by hunger or thirst. Whatever occurs in the past or future, in the three worlds, becomes known to him. (329)

All that becomes directly perceived by him, and omniscience arises. With respect to inner time, there comes knowledge and true discernment. (330)

All this, together with its many parts, has been explained; understand it. Thus ends the seventh chapter of the Svācchanda Tantra. (331)

ॐ

www.ingramcontent.com/pod-product-compliance
Lightning Source LLC
LaVergne TN
LVHW010600100826
845148LV00014B/2785

* 9 7 8 9 6 5 9 3 3 4 4 0 7 *